THE
Hardness
FACTOR™

THE
Hardness
FACTOR™

How to Achieve Your Best Health and Sexual Fitness at Any Age

STEVEN LAMM, M.D.

with **GERALD SECOR COUZENS**

HarperCollins*Publishers*

This book is written as a source of information only. The information contained in this book should by no means be considered a substitute for the advice of a qualified medical professional, who should always be consulted before beginning any new diet, exercise, or health program.

All efforts have been made to ensure the accuracy of the information contained in this book as of the date published. The author and the publisher expressly disclaim responsibility for any adverse effects arising from the use or application of the information contained herein.

HarperCollins books may be purchased for educational, business, or sales promotional use. For information, please write: Special Markets Department, HarperCollins Publishers, 10 East 53rd Street, New York, NY 10022.

FIRST EDITION

The Hardness Factor™ is a registered trademark of Jeff Stone Again LTD.

A NEW BRAND IDEA

JEFF STONE AGAIN LTD.
jeffstoneagain@mac.com
ILLUSTRATIONS BY JONNY COHEN
EXERCISE REGIME BY JANA ANGELAKIS
DESIGNED BY LUCY ALBANESE

Printed on acid-free paper

Library of Congress Cataloging-in-Publication Data
is available upon request.

ISBN-10: 0-06-075551-2
ISBN-13: 978-0-06-075551-5

05 06 07 08 09 ❖/RRD 10 9 8 7 6 5 4 3 2 1

To my beautiful wife, Kiki,
whose love nourishes and supports me.
To my mother, Lucy, whose vitality inspires me.
And to my five loving children,
David, Suzanne, Alexandra, Morgan, and Owen.

STEVEN LAMM, M.D.

To Elisa, Gerald, Dominic, Mary, and Rose,
my love and appreciation forever.
To F.X.M., who kept it real.

GERALD SECOR COUZENS

To the world, hello.
Jonny Cohen

Acknowledgments

This book would not have been possible without the experience and assistance of many people. We would like to thank those colleagues, patients, friends, and family members who have helped us the most.

Dr. Mariano Rosselló, the innovative urologist from Mallorca who invented the Digital Inflection Rigidometer; his daughter, Anabel Rosselló, who came to New York and first assisted us with our studies; and Marc Cohen, M.D., the urologist and Napa Valley vintner who first put us in touch with the Rosselló family.

The nascent field of male sexual medicine has been advanced through the efforts and innovations of several key urologists. We give special thanks to Dr. Irwin Goldstein and Dr. Ridwan Shabsigh for their research and scientific breakthroughs, and to Dr. Lawrence Hakim for his medical expertise and good humor.

Thanks to Victor Ferrari and Frank Assuma of Horphag Research, Mel Rich of Pinnacle, and Jerry Kay of the Integrated BioPharma, who helped with our studies. Thanks also to James and Loren Ridinger, Marty Weissman, and Joe Bolyard from Market America.

We would also like to thank Paul Johnson, Levitra brand manager for GlaxoSmithKline, and Dawn Bradway, the associate director of Medical

Science for Bayer, who understood the importance of erection quality and hardness, and that hardness does matter. We also want to thank Chad Royer, the Lilly marketing director for Cialis, who champions the importance of male sexual health and the link between biology and intimacy.

Several years ago, I was offered a unique opportunity to reach a women's television market about important men's health issues. Many thanks to Barbara Walters and Bill Geddie for providing me with this important forum on *The View,* the Emmy Award–winning daytime show. My work is made much easier thanks to *The View* co-hosts Meredith Vieira, Star Jones Reynolds, Joy Behar, and Elisabeth Hasselbeck. It's the Emmy Award–winning director, Mark Gentile, Sue Solomon and producers Patrick Ignozzi and Dana Goodman, who help make it all look so easy.

We acknowledge with deep gratitude the valuable help of these people who contributed information to the book: Elisa Michel, Rosemary Michel, and Matthew Michel.

We would also like to thank David Emile, owner of Beacon Restaurant, and his partner, chef-owner Waldy Malouf, for the delicious recipes and culinary insights; Jonny Cohen for his humorous look at life; and Jana Angelakis, Olympic athlete and fitness expert, for her exercise expertise.

We would like to thank Bo Dietel, Ted Shields, and his late brother, Tim, for understanding the relationship between heart health, omega 3s, and hardness, and their efforts in helping spread this important message.

Thanks are in order for Billy Norwich, who offered his critical eye and constant support and review throughout the writing process, while Tana Kokol helped with her nutrition suggestions.

Cathy Hemming initially saw this as an important book and championed it throughout HarperCollins, and it was Susan Weinberg's focus and determination that helped this book come to life. David Hirshey, our indefatigable editor; Michael Solomon, our book, style, and taste guide; and Nick Trautwein, David's associate editor, offered guidance, support, and high levels of patience as the book came together. We also thank Lucy Albanese for creating such a beautifully designed book. And a special thanks to Carrie Kania for her enthusiasm in making sure the message of men's health reaches the widest audience possible. For that, and much more, we are indebted.

And finally, we would like to thank Jeff Stone, a staunch ally and friend who believed in this project right from the start, as he sat in my office one hot summer afternoon a long time ago and pondered.

Steven Lamm, M.D.
Gerald Secor Couzens
NEW YORK, N.Y.
JANUARY 2005

Contents

Part Two

The Hardness Factor Six-Week Program
Hard Is Good—Harder Is Better

Part **Three**

Hardness for Life
(or at Least Through Friday Night)

Appendices

SEX is important to a healthy man. _The Hardness Factor_ is, first and foremost, a health book. When you are physically and emotionally healthy, your penis is hard when you are aroused. This book is also about the essence of _maleness_ and how masculinity is intimately bound up in the idea of _hardness_ and its relation to the penis. And yes, it is politically correct to admit that you have a penis and that it does get hard.

Let's face it, men need to be hard. Not only is much of our self-image dependent on it, but so too is the creation of life. So much that is important in our life flows from this notion of hardness. Men's sexual identity is intimately linked to this fragile appendage that becomes engorged—_how_ engorged is the reason behind this book.

The Hardness Factor is about a new definition of maleness. In the last forty years, the old chauvinistic notions of male superiority have been properly discarded as hurtful relics of the past. Eliminating this old baggage is well deserved. Nevertheless, in jettisoning those stereotypes, I believe, some important and positive aspects of being a man have been lost or marginalized.

The ideas of self-sufficiency, physical strength, and confidence—a man's mental hardness as well as his physical hardness—are vital parts of being a man. Moreover, a crucial aspect of male hardness is the strength of his erection. When the penis is hard, life is good. When hardness diminishes, so does a man's health and his innate sense of who he is.

For all of us, there comes a time when there is a change in penile hardness. The dependability of an erection wavers—this is a physical reality. There are important medical and psychological implications that often come with these changes—imperceptible changes. I am talking about subtle changes that occur in every man, more slowly in healthy, younger men, more precipitately in those who have ignored their health or are affected by certain illnesses.

> 66 When the penis is hard, life is good. When hardness diminishes, so does a man's health and his innate sense of who he is.

We are all sexual beings and sex is an essential part of who we are. The fact that you are reading these words shows that you take erections, sex, and health very seriously. Unfortunately, most young men (and women) in this country fail to understand what links the three.

Men are an endangered species. We are dying from a variety of diseases that could easily have been prevented had they been addressed much earlier. We are dying from cardiovascular disease, our number one killer. We die of cancers (particularly of the prostate and colon) that have either metastasized or were detected too late. We die from the effects of depression and bipolar disorder, which often result in fatal heart attacks and suicide as we age. In essence, we are dying of a slew of disorders that can be prevented. Moreover, men are extremely slow to react when it comes to our own health and well-being.

What is it going to take to change this particular male trait of medical denial? It has always been very clear to me that men need some kind of motivating force to bring about positive health changes. And when you think of men and think of motivation, I think of only one thing: sex.

In just the past decade, researchers have made the all-important link between sexual activity and good health. When a man's blood vessels are healthy and "elastic," his heart and brain are functioning well—and his erections are rock hard.

When his neural connections are firing and nitric oxide is being released in great abundance throughout his body, his cognition is high—and his erections are rock hard. When testosterone levels are normal and weight is controlled, he has the ability to train most effectively—have a healthy, trim body—and his erections are rock hard. Once men start to connect the dots, once they fully understand that good health and a hard erection are synonymous, they will begin to take better care of themselves.

Men grow up appreciating that a part of their anatomy changes in a cyclical fashion throughout the day, starting with erections in the morning. They awaken from a deep sleep with an erection that holds the covers inches away from their body. Most don't have to work to have an erection; one may appear at the oddest moments. As they grow older, however, they're somewhat perturbed by the lack of these spontaneous erections. They no longer experience them when they're sitting around, nor do they become aroused at the slightest sexual thought, as they did when they were teenagers.

> 66 Men are an endangered species.

Many men are disturbed that even with extensive sexual stimulation, erections are often less hard and reliable. This confuses them. Some are ashamed that they can no longer get hard, or that they are not quite so hard as they used to be. A part of them has changed, for some reason they can't understand. The way many choose to deal with it is to ignore it. It's a guy thing—denial. It might get better, they think. Eventually. Unfortunately, for some, *eventually* can stretch out over a period of years until it turns into never.

Here is a typical example from my case file of male medical ignorance.

BEN, age 28—Soft smoke

Ben, a handsome 28-year-old insurance broker, came in recently with a complaint of bronchitis. He had waited until he was so sick that he had thrown his back out from all of his coughing. His yellowed index finger was a none-too-subtle tip-off to his two-pack-a-day smoking habit. I examined him and treated him for his infection. Before leaving, however, I also urged him to throw away his cigarettes for good.

"Oh, yeah, so I won't get cancer," he said.

"No, because you're going to have problems getting a hard erection," I told him. "If you don't have problems already. I want you to stop smoking now and make changes at a time in your life when sexual performance is still very relevant. I know that the fear of cancer in your 50s and 60s is not a powerful enough factor—two decades seems too far away. However, I do know that performance and a softening erection are even more realistic fears."

Ben sat up straight in his chair. "I had no idea smoking could have been a cause," he said. Ben admitted that his erections had not been so hard as he once remembered. He had chalked it up to aging—after all he wasn't 17 anymore—a self-protective form of delusion. I chalked it up to cigarettes. He left the office that afternoon with several sample boxes of nicotine patches.

Once a man realizes that smoking damages his hardness, he is given a powerful motivating force for change. The same goes for men with hypertension, the "silent killer." This ailment is not only about having a heart attack or stroke at some unforeseen point in the future. Rather, it's also about weak and progressively weaker erections: right now. As in today.

When I tell a man that obesity is not just about being thirty or more pounds more than an ideal weight for his age and height, but that it affects hardness and influences his ability to obtain and sustain an erection suitable for penetration—and will do so until he loses some weight—he listens carefully. He now has real motivation.

When a man hears that continually monitoring and regulating blood sugar to keep his diabetes under control means that his erections will be strong at night, I have his full attention.

Over the years, I have found that once men come to understand that their hardness depends on taking better care of themselves, they become much better patients. They take a more proactive stance when it comes to their health because they comprehend the far-reaching effects of the alternative.

The Hardness Factor is a book about the preservation and enhancement of a man's erections. If he chooses not to preserve and enhance, but instead ignore his health, he will have to restore sexual function at some point in the future—guaranteed. And that may entail anything from prescription drugs and injections to penile implant surgery. Believe me: preserving and enhancing are much easier than restoring.

This is a book that will tell you how your penis works and what it takes to attain a firm, hard erection—at any age. And no matter how hard your erection is presently, I can help you make it even harder. My message to all men is basic and direct: When you are able to have a hard erection every time, you are generally in the best possible health.

The ability to have truly satisfying sex depends, in great part, on your overall physical condition. When you are fit, you are also confident and happy with your body. Your hard erection—and muscular body that is equally hard—allows you to fully partake in vigorous and prolonged lovemaking with your partner. Moreover, when your partner is confident of your hardness, total focus during lovemaking can be placed on creating intimacy and experiencing and giving pleasure.

As you read *The Hardness Factor*, you will come to see the pivotal role a hard erection plays in physical and psychological health. *The Hardness Factor* is as much about learning what not to do as it is about learning what to do. Just as good lifestyle choices will keep you young and rejuvenate your physical and mental states to a degree you never dreamed possible, so too can poor lifestyle choices damage your health.

This knowledge can change your entire life, as it has for me and many of my patients. By following my suggestions, I assure you that a man can be healthy, active, and hard well into his 70s and beyond. At its very core, *The Hardness Factor* is a detailed health program. What you learn from this book will answer so many questions about erections, sexual frequency, masturbation, premature ejaculation, performance anxiety, and partner satisfaction. Sensuality is taken to a new level. Sex is more pleasurable. Intimacy is enhanced. You will enjoy life much more.

Your partner will, too. What condition do you know in which a positive change in a person's health enhances the health of his partner as well? If you lose weight, your partner doesn't lose weight. If you lower your cholesterol or reduce your blood pressure, you don't expect your partner's cholesterol or blood pressure to drop.

> 66 Researchers have just reported that when a man is hard and healthy and enjoying regular sex, he also enhances the performance and sexual satisfaction of his partner.

However, researchers have just reported that when a man is hard and healthy and enjoying regular sex, he also enhances the performance and sexual satisfaction of his partner.

As a practicing internist and a researcher for the past decade, I have long examined the effects of sexual medicine. I am increasingly impressed by how much we now have at hand to maintain hardness and also by how little we have taken advantage of that knowledge. It is time we put these newly found discoveries to work for the sake of overall health.

When I was in medical school more than twenty-five years ago, we were taught that hardness problems were psychological, that they were "all in your head." We now know that that simply is not true—and we have ways to reverse many of those problems. The good news I will be offering in *The Hardness Factor* is based on the recent explosive growth in sexual medicine that started after the release of Viagra, the pharmaceutical blockbuster, in

1998. We now understand that increasing blood flow to the penis strengthens erections and enhances the function of that vital organ. I guarantee that this new medical knowledge will not only change a man's life, but it could save that life as well.

As a doctor who counsels and treats men and women with sexual concerns, I will guide you through my special program of enhancement and describe the lifestyle changes that I want you to make. I will offer delicious food selections to heighten your taste sensation and also aid in increasing your hardness. I will describe a variety of exercises I want you to try that will bolster your mobility, strength, flexibility, and endurance—and make sex even more pleasurable.

> 66 You may discover that the erection you save may also save your companion's life.

Using such nutritional powerhouses as Pycnogenol, L-arginine, omega-3 fatty acids, horny goat weed, and a host of antioxidant supplements, men can prevent and reverse most hardness problems. I will also detail what prescription medications you may need to take—or not need at all.

If you take advantage of this knowledge and put into action a few simple measures I recommend, you can almost certainly optimize your hardness, enhance your relationship with your significant other, and lengthen your active years.

Although this is a book for men who clearly need to understand the relationship between sexual health and overall health, perhaps you are a girlfriend, a wife, or a male partner in a relationship and you're concerned about what's really going on. Well, this book is written for you, too. It is packed with all the practical, research-based information you have been longing for and it will help you understand the central role of an erection in a man's being so you will understand the changes that may occur over time. You may discover that the erection you save may also save your companion's life.

Overall, my hope is that *The Hardness Factor* will help everyone understand more about themselves as sexual beings and healthy individuals who want a long and vital life. This book offers real lifestyle suggestions that will rejuvenate you, help you gain control over your health—and your erections—and pave the way to feeling confident and powerful into the upcoming years. That is the reason for my book. In the following chapters, read and make the right choices in caring for your body as you begin your journey toward maintaining your hardness and health for life. Now, let's get started. And remember, hard is good; harder is better.

Be well.
Dr. Steven Lamm

Part One

THE MENTAL AND PHYSICAL ASPECTS OF HARDNESS

66*Am I hard enough*
Am I rough enough
Am I rich enough
I'm not too blind to see

"Beast of Burden,"
The Rolling Stones

WHAT IS THE HARDNESS FACTOR?

DEGREES OF HARDNESS ≻ ≻ ≻ ≻ ≻ ≻ ≻ ≻ ≻ ≻ ≻ ≻ ≻

Aman may think he's best friends with his penis, but how well does he really know it? Few are aware that there are degrees of penile hardness. Fewer still know what "normal" hardness is. Age, exercise, diet, and stress can affect a man's erectile quality (EQ)— even men in their early 20s, all full of testosterone, the source of masculinity and hardness, sometimes fail to achieve an erection. More worrisome is that men 40 years of age or older have a 50 percent chance of getting and maintaining an erection. Those numbers rise exponentially as the decades increase. But the good news is that all these hardness factors are within a man's control.

How Dependable Is Your Penis?

BILL, age 31—Hard as a rock?

My answering service called early one Monday morning to say that Bill had already called twice, each time with the message that he had to see me first thing that morning. Bill was 31, an in-demand studio guitarist, whose first CD had just been released by a major label. I was a bit surprised that he would be calling since I had just given him a complete medical work-up a month earlier as part of a life insurance policy he was applying for. He was in very good mental health, and I recalled having congratulated this ardent "meat and potatoes" guy on good cholesterol numbers.

When Bill came in, he appeared nervous and agitated, and somewhat sheepish. He's a handsome, fit guy with a thick mustache flecked with gray that offsets his completely shaved head. I ushered him into my office and he was about to say something when he noticed that my door was not completely shut. He popped out of his chair, closed it firmly, and then sat down again.

"I've got a problem that's driving me nuts, which is why I need to see you," he said. "It concerns a woman who's important in my life. No, actually that's not really true. It's not about the woman at all. It's about me." He looked down at his feet, obviously embarrassed. "Well, to be more precise, it's about my penis. I need help. Fast. I need one of those six-packs of Viagra."

"All right, Bill, slow down," I said. "Why do you think you need Viagra?"

"Karen is flying in next month from Santa Barbara," he said. "And I'm really crazy about her. But if I have another awkward moment like I did the last time and can't maintain my erection and hold my own in bed, I know I'll be deleted from her speed dial. She's not going to give me another chance. I have such anxiety over this that I'm certain I'm not gonna be able to get it up."

I asked Bill if he was having any problems getting the initial erection. He seemed perplexed by the question. "I can get an erection," he said. "In fact, as soon as I see her, I'm hard as a rock." He paused for a moment. "It's not that I'm having problems there. It's just that my erection seems softer once we get going. It seems to disappear for a while when we're getting hot and heavy, and it's a lot of work to get it back. It's really annoying and, to tell you the truth, it's becoming a big deal for me."

"First of all," I told Bill, "this is not uncommon, so I don't want you to panic. You'd be surprised how many guys have crises of confidence. You're not alone there, but," I went on, "you have to understand that penises are temperamental and too often we allow ourselves to be judged by them. That naturally puts a lot of pressure on us to perform. One day can be great, the next day a complete horror show. But yours is a problem that I can definitely help you with."

"You can help guys with limp dicks?" Bill asked.

"Actually, you don't have a limp dick, Bill," I said. "You just aren't as hard as you want to be. You know, sometimes it's amazing that any of us manage to have erections at all. These are true, mind-body events connected with highly-tuned physiological workings. It's all part of what I call the Hardness Factor.

> 66 Sometimes it's amazing that any of us manage to have erections at all. These are true, mind-body events connected with highly-tuned physiological workings.

"The Hardness Factor is not only about having erections, but about feeling more confident about your erections, more sure of yourself as a sexual person—the surprise is that it's also about your health. For the past couple of years, I have been slowly developing a program to help enhance erectile hardness. I've conducted clinical studies that have never been done before to assess what works and what doesn't: herbal products, prescription drugs, exercise, you name it. The Six-Week Program I've developed ensures that you can confidently expect to maintain a hard erection during lovemaking."

I asked Bill if he would like to have something that would give him the confidence that he could perform when Karen arrived. What Bill required was something that would produce dramatic results in a very short time.

His face brightened, and he appeared somewhat relieved. "Great. You are going to give me the Viagra?"

"You actually don't need prescription drugs," I told him. "You already get erections. I'm sure that if I ran one of my clinical tests on you, you would score very high for hardness."

Bill was puzzled. "Are you down on the medications?" he wanted to know. "I thought Viagra was supposed to be great."

"Viagra, Cialis, and Levitra are great for those men who really need the drugs," I explained. "I can give you whichever medication you need. You just take any of these pills and fifteen minutes later, you will be ready for sex. The fact that we have these drugs is a wonderful thing, and I'm certainly not hesitant in prescribing them. But I reserve them for men who really need to use them in order to get an erection. And luckily, you're not one of them.

"You're young and healthy, and my assessment is that your problem is a minor condition that's developed because of stress. I've got something better that will improve your confidence, your hardness, and your health."

I reached for a folder on the shelf behind my desk. "Let me give you this copy of my program," I said, handing him the sheaf of pages that detailed how I wanted him to eat, drink, exercise, and sleep over the next six weeks.

"Not only will it improve your heart and muscles, but I guarantee that it will help strengthen your erections as well. As you will see," I said, "there are certain foods that I want you to eat. These foods contain a host of prosexual nutrients that will help increase hardness by increasing blood flow."

I also wanted Bill to take an herbal product that would maintain his libido despite the heightened anxiety he had about his upcoming performance. Tension is a frequent suppressor of libido, I told him, and I gave him a container of pills. "Take these daily," I said, "and within two days you may end up with vivid sexual dreams like you've never had before. I want you to take an extra dose shortly before any expected sexual encounter with Karen."

I also suggested that he take another supplement, what one of my patients calls his "penis vitamins." This natural product contains antioxidants and a special amino acid that prepares the blood vessels for optimal blood delivery and maximum hardness.

"Finally," I said to Bill, "I want you to perform certain exercises twice daily that increase the strength in key muscles involved in sex, and also enhance blood flow to the groin area."

Bill quickly scanned the pages I had handed him about the program, and then looked up. "Just doing these things will make that big a difference in bed?" he wanted to know.

I nodded. "And here's why: Viagra, Levitra, and Cialis offer instantaneous solutions. Those pills will give you an erection. Period. But I'm offering you something much more than those prescription drugs can give you. By following this program, you will be instrumental in maintaining and sustaining the erection. And that's what is going to restore your confidence and reaffirm your masculinity. It's going to put the Hardness Factor under your total control once again."

Bill thanked me for my help. "I hope this works," he said as he got up to leave. "It's so lousy feeling this way because it affects everything I do."

TO BE CONTINUED ▶

SO WHAT *IS* THE HARDNESS FACTOR?

Let's be clear: Erections are important to men. It is part of how we define our identities. This is true for young men, old men, men who have had a heart attack, men who are blind, and men who have diabetes or other chronic ailments. And no matter how talented a man may feel he is in bed, he defines sex by his erection, by its strength and hardness. This is what I call the Hardness Factor. The harder the erection, the healthier the man. Both men and their partners need a better understanding of the factors that affect hardness.

> 66 The harder the erection, the healthier the man.

Naturally, because men want to be hard, many are afraid of losing their hardness. And just as we need glasses to enhance our vision as we get older, stretch and work out to maintain flexibility, walk regularly to maintain lung capacity, so too must steps be taken to enhance and maintain hardness.

The Hardness Factor is also about gaining and maintaining sexual fitness. But what is sexual fitness? Does that mean having sex a certain number of times per week? Or is it more about having a healthy attitude about sex? My definition of sexual fitness is straightforward: being in great sexual shape—having a healthy body, a strong libido, and the ability to be as hard as you possibly can.

Moreover, maintaining the Hardness Factor is a proactive way of living. When you understand its basic concepts, you realize how sexuality is a window into general health—that the hardness of the penis is the best indicator of general health and how by staying fit a man can enjoy being a male as long as he lives.

The bottom line: After following the Hardness Factor Program, men will be in the best sexual shape of their lives, enjoy better sex that lasts longer, and live healthier lives.

THE NEW PROMISE OF SEXUAL MEDICINE

Men and their partners are often confused when it comes to hardness. That's because penile hardness is such a wildly individualized, yet variable trait that can change based on the hour, day, and time of the year. Hardness can also be different before and after meals. It's affected by how much exercise a man performs, how much alcohol he imbibes, the amount of stress in his life, and what medications he takes, as well as when he takes them. I've seen too many men thrown wildly off course by not understanding what hardness means, what affects it, and what is necessary to maintain it. Erections don't just happen—everything impacts hardness. A cold. Whether or not the favorite team wins. A tough day at work or a sick family member.

In addition to taking care of patients in my busy Manhattan medical practice, I appear regularly on *The View* as one of the "in-house doctors" to discuss important medical issues with Barbara Walters and her four lovely cohorts. What I like so much about *The View* is the fact that this Emmy Award–winning program affords me the opportunity to be in a women's world filled with their countless questions about men.

I am also an assistant clinical professor of internal medicine at NYU School of Medicine where I teach our future doctors, and I regularly lecture nationwide about sexual medicine issues. I am a member of the North American Society for Sexual Medicine. It was my book *The Virility Solution*—which was published the same month in 1998 that the FDA approved Viagra—that heralded this exciting new era of men's sexual medicine.

But what is sexual medicine? Yes, there is the preventive dimension, which alerts people to be more careful and sexually aware about their health. But it's not just about sexually transmitted diseases. What I have found to be the more exciting area (and the one that has changed so radically in the past few years) is linked to the aspects of sexual medicine brought on by the introduction of Viagra. This one erection drug has triggered the same sort of revolution in sexual medicine as Prozac did in the world of psychiatry and mental health.

❝ Viagra has triggered the same sort of revolution in sexual medicine as Prozac did in the world of psychiatry and mental health.

Psychologists and psychiatrists would be the first to tell you that the use of this psychopharmaceutical helps a tremendous number of people with depression, but it is the combination of medical therapy and counseling that is essential in order to elicit a cure. So true with Viagra. Our society always wants to believe in cures by the "magic" pill, but I have found from my years of experience in treating psychiatric and sexual issues that it is even better if a patient never has to take medication.

What excites me about this era of sexual medicine is that it has brought about a new awareness of the completely interrelated aspects of mind and body. We now know, for example, that by taking care of your overall health, you will also be taking care of your sexual health. It is this knowledge that has led me to develop a series of non-pharmacological treatments that form the basis of the Hardness Factor Six-Week Program.

VIAGRA: THE PILL THAT STARTED IT ALL

Viagra was introduced in 1998, initiating a medical revolution that very slowly turned into a massive culture shift. Not since the introduction of the Pill fifty years ago has something so important to sexuality made its debut. All in all, this little blue 50-mg pill has been one of the most significant medical breakthroughs, not only because it can restore hardness, but because it made possible the important dialogue that now allows all men to talk openly about their sexual dysfunction concerns.

This dialogue can now occur between doctor and doctor; between men and their doctors; between men and their partners; between friends. What this new, open discussion has done is demonstrate yet again how important one's sexual identity is to who you think you are, the way you view yourself, and the way you understand yourself.

As one of the principal investigators of an erection medication in a lengthy FDA study, I not only gained firsthand knowledge about these new drugs, but more important, I had a chance to talk to dozens of men and their partners about the impact of hardness on their lives. My book *The Virility Solution* was a result of this important clinical research.

In the intervening years, I have dispensed thousands of prescriptions for erection-enhancing drugs, and what has really

---

*F**rom Heart to Hard***

In the early 1990s, scientists at the Pfizer laboratory in Sandwich, England, conducting a drug study with an experimental heart medication were distressed to find that the drug was not increasing blood flow to the heart as well as had been expected. However, when men in the study were reluctant to return their leftover drugs at the end of the study because they said that it triggered powerful erections, the scientists decided to shift their study focus. Viagra, the former heart drug, received FDA approval several years later as the first prescription hardness drug and went on to become one of the biggest-selling drugs in history.

impressed me the most is how restorative—in a variety of ways—these drugs can be. I was initially thankful to be able to take care of men, and I was happy to watch how the medicine rejuvenated them and changed their lives. Sometimes men were encouraged enough that they started to exercise again and get in better physical shape. Others found that the restoration of their sex lives helped relieve their depressive symptoms. A man walking by his mirror with a full erection is one of the best antidepressants we have.

But what had men done to put themselves in a position where they needed these erection drugs? There had to be a way, I felt, to protect and preserve their hardness so that they never reached the point where they needed restoration.

THE GENESIS OF THE HARDNESS FACTOR

I was becoming increasingly concerned and frustrated about the level of denial so many of my patients had about their sexual health. To begin with, men rarely wanted to talk about their overall health. When they did come in for an appointment, talking about sexual problems was something they danced around as best they could. I was frustrated because they were ignoring the all-important link between their sexual health and their general health.

Even more frustrating was when a man came in for a visit, assumed he was having an erection problem, and therefore wanted me to immediately write a prescription for the "little blue pill." By using an erection drug when it is unneeded, the underlying lifestyle problems that can be reversed through modest changes in diet, physical activity, and supplements are overlooked.

From years of experience, I had already created a profile in my mind of the men who were likely to be experiencing hardness problems. They were shocked and embarrassed when asked the question point-blank: When did you first notice you were having erection difficulties? A few years ago, as yet another man walked out of my office with a prescription for Viagra, I had an epiphany. I asked this of myself: Why does a man have to get so sick in order to regain some of his former hardness? Does he really have to be sick to want optimum health and hardness?

GETTING IN SHAPE FOR SEX

Why can't men be in shape for sex their entire lives? What if they just stayed hard and well their whole lives? Intuitively, I knew this was possible. I certainly had enough patients—many older than 60—who were physically active and sexually fit. From my own ongoing exercise and hardness studies, I have found that many of the declines in hardness often attributed to age are actually the result of sedentary living and poor nutrition.

> 66 Why can't men be in shape for sex their entire lives?

My point is that hardness problems, even erectile dysfunction, are not inevitable, nor will every man over the age of 50 need Viagra, Cialis, or Levitra. Regular exercise boosts sexual performance, while inactivity increases men's risk of erectile dysfunction, a condition we now commonly call ED.

If I have learned one thing about my patients, it is this: they respond to numbers. They know their body weight, body fat percentage, blood pressure, cholesterol, and PSA levels. Patients interested in preventive measures use all of these numbers to make dramatic and important lifestyle changes. Others, however, need a jolt to make them take action.

Thanks to a new diagnostic device, I am now able to provide men with a figure that neither they nor 99.9 percent of the doctors in the world have ever seen before. It is a number guaranteed to make men sit up and listen very attentively. It is the number that tells me how hard their penis is—the Hardness Factor.

This number comes from a simple, five-second test that measures the strength of an erection. The results of this test have far greater implications than a mere satisfying sex life. A low hardness factor number, for example, could signal undetected heart disease, diabetes, hypertension, obesity, sleep apnea, and many other important health issues. I have found that when it comes to sexual fitness, when a man's diet is poor and exercise is limited, there is no better way to get men on track than by using the Digital Inflection Rigidometer (DIR). I will explain more about this revolutionary device later on.

SEX IS A MEASURE OF A MAN'S HEALTH

According to a new study of 2,400 men from researchers at the University of Bristol in England, men who reported three or more orgasms per week enjoyed a 50 percent reduction in heart attacks and strokes compared to those who have sex less often.

On the surface, it looks as though the principal message of this study is that having sex reduces the incidence of heart attack and stroke and lets you live longer. In fact, just the opposite is true: being healthy allows you to have sex as much as you want. Having sex three times a week serves as an important marker that you are healthy and in good physical shape—you're certainly more sexually fit than people who can't have sex three times a week.

Beyond that, the strength of a man's erection—his hardness—is the true barometer of his overall health. I first started realizing this years ago when I noted the powerful and unmistakable link between failing erections and common medical ailments, including obesity, high cholesterol levels, hypertension, depression, sleep disorders, diabetes, and heart disease.

In treating men with these chronic complaints, it had become almost routine that by the second or third office visit, the patients began describing sexual issues that were

> **66** Having sex three times a week serves as an important marker that you are healthy and in good physical shape.

actually bothering them more than the original medical complaint. The reason for their prior reluctance in seeking help was that they just felt they had no one they could speak to who would completely understand their complaints.

I was different, they said. Not only was I a good listener, but I also had workable solutions. It became clear to me that the quality of a man's erection was damaged by more than just chronic illness. There was a strong psychological component to sex as well, and I routinely began examining the psychosocial history of my patients. Job problems, money worries, relationship issues, and deaths in the family typically created serious hardness issues for many, exacerbating preexisting problems even more.

> 66 The strength of a man's erection is the true barometer of his overall health.

OUR MEDICATED SOCIETY—A HARDNESS FACTOR

Our modern world is one of anxiety, economic worries, poor diet and exercise regimens, and long hours at work; we also live in a highly medicated society. There is now growing awareness of depression as a real health condition that—like such diseases as cancer, diabetes, and heart disease—is highly prevalent. Since 1996, doctor visits for depression have increased by more than a third, and related drug prescriptions have risen 63 percent.

Many men of all ages now take Prozac, Zoloft, Paxil, Depakote, and a variety of other antidepressants, as well as a slew of medications for treating everything from hypertension and obesity to diabetes and heart problems. Most, if not all, of these drugs affect hardness, with as many as 33 to 40 percent of patients who take them going on to develop some degree of sexual dysfunction. The sexual side effects can become so pronounced for some that it's now estimated that almost 90 percent of depressed patients who develop sexual problems consequently stop taking their antidepressants too soon, which can put them at a risk for relapse of depression. (For a complete listing of medications with hardness side effects, please see *thehardnessfactor.com*.)

THE BIG LIE: ONLY OLD MEN LIMP INTO THAT GOOD NIGHT

The prevailing myth is that younger men are immune to hardness concerns. I've got sobering news for you: they're not.

As I began to look closer at my younger patients, men in their 20s and early 30s, I found that many were not completely satisfied with the quality, frequency, and overall hardness of their erections. There were performance anxiety issues. Young men wanted to know why they couldn't always get hard after a night of drinking. Why was marijuana such a downer and Ecstasy such an erection killer? Many complained of hardness that showed up quickly and left even quicker—rapid ejaculation is now the nomenclature for what is also called premature ejaculation—and how this embarrassed them. Putting on a condom, especially when they were with a new partner, was a major issue and a definite hardness impediment.

Many men wanted to know how they could be "ready and primed" for the big weekend date. Right or wrong, men compete, especially with themselves; most of all, they wanted the individual confidence to score a 10, or at the very least, not embarrass themselves in the act of sex.

This crisis of confidence reminded me of a similar phenomenon young women experienced thirty or forty years ago when they read Dr. Alex Comfort's *The Joy of Sex* or *The Sensuous Woman* by "J" so as not to appear foolish to their partners. But now, programs such as *Sex and the City* show women's empowerment, a development of women's sophistication humorously juxtaposed with the lack of sophistication in their male companions. And in this social paradigm shift, it's now young men who are concerned with being less than adequate. We are a society that grades ability, and the penis—in men of all ages—is likewise scrutinized.

Young men are developing serious relationships and trying to find out who they are and what it is they want from life. Many are confused and their questions are endless. Their muddled ideas and misconceptions about sex and hardness have left them vulnerable. They didn't feel like themselves, so they asked me to help. Their pleas only made me more determined to find workable solutions. In a world of significant empowerment for women, hardness really matters for men.

HARDNESS FACT: IT'S THE ERECTION QUALITY NUMBERS THAT ARE FALLING

When it comes to erectile problems, men are often surprised to discover that they are no different from other men, that their concerns are shared by many, and that, unfortunately, when it comes to serious dysfunctions, their numbers are growing.

Thanks to the introduction of Viagra, Cialis, and Levitra, there is now a greater awareness of erection quality. When a man doesn't pay attention to his erection quality (EQ), the end result will be erectile dysfunction (ED). ED is defined as the consistent or recurrent inability to obtain or maintain a penile erection sufficient for sexual performance. It's now estimated that 34 percent of all American men ages 40 to 70—about 20 million men—suffer from some significant level of ED. Unfortunately, most of them—about 80 percent according to researchers at Pfizer Inc. (the makers of Viagra)—never seek treatment. That means that millions of men are unfulfilled in the sexual arena, and a good many of these men are living lives of quiet desperation.

> 66 34 percent of all American men ages 40 to 70—about 20 million men—suffer from some significant level of ED.

HOW HARD IS YOUR PENIS?

I became an expert on male sexual problems partly because I'm a man, but mainly from being an internal medicine specialist with a powerful curiosity for how and why things work and why they become impaired or simply fail to function. Even as I was involved in research studies and read about the purported benefits of herbal supplements, something really changed and made me start taking sexual medicine seriously.

In my past FDA-sanctioned studies with the erection drugs Viagra and Vasomax, I relied solely on the International Index of Erectile Function, a self-scoring questionnaire of fifteen questions men would use before and after treatment for their dysfunction. After a while, it became very clear to me that the IIEF had a major flaw—it was subjective and anecdotal. With the stroke of a pencil, embarrassed subjects could easily elevate their hardness, lying to themselves as well as to researchers. However, all that changed the day that I first used the Digital Inflection Rigidometer.

Several years ago, I was introduced to Dr. Mariano Rosselló, a remarkable Spanish urologist from Mallorca. What Dr. Rosselló had invented in his home workshop was the DIR, a compact, hand-held, computerized device that could accurately measure the hardness of an erection. Dr. Rosselló had been using the device to measure hardness in older men with ED before and after prostate cancer surgery in order to determine the progression of their penetration capacity. I immediately saw the usefulness of his DIR for measuring the hardness of younger, healthier men.

My goal was to find out if men were performing at optimal hardness levels, and if not, why? Finally, I had a device that offered me, well, hard evidence about the state of a man's overall health. I am now one of a handful of researchers and specialists in the United States who have this innovative research device.

To obtain a DIR reading, all a man has to do is get an erection, press the device gently against the tip of his erect penis until it buckles, and then hold it there for five seconds. This is all it takes to register a man's hardness and his ability to penetrate. Measurements of his hardness in grams of pressure are obtained and immediately stored on a computer chip. Back in my office, I can download all the information about the man's erection capabilities and note how much room there is for improvement.

In the past several years, I have used the DIR and tested the hardness of hundreds of men, ranging in age from 18 to 75. I can now quantify hardness just as easily as I can use a blood test to quantify elevated cholesterol, diabetes, or hypertension. With the DIR, I now have a scientific evidence-based way to measure the reality and success of the Hardness Factor.

HOW HARD IS HARD—THE DIR NUMBERS

400 grams or less > Indicates the penis is limp—like string—and there may be possible underlying medical problems causing this. Intercourse is difficult at best. There needs to be an earnest discussion with the doctor about making serious changes in a number of possible hardness risk factors.

500–600 grams > A man is borderline hard. He's hard for a while, soft, and then hard. He needs the Hardness Factor Six-Week Program to raise his score to consistently healthier and harder levels.

1,000 grams > Very good hardness—imagine a piece of oak—and a mark every healthy man should be able to achieve.

1,500–2,000 grams > The man is extremely healthy. Imagine a steel beam for an erection.

2,000+ grams > Titanium. It is understood that the man is in excellent health, that he does not smoke or drink to excess, and gets plenty of rest—and is probably 15 years old.

A MEASURE OF A MAN—IT'S NOT IN INCHES

I could present to those seemingly healthy young men—who began exercising and taking the supplements I recommended in the Hardness Factor

Six-Week Program—with "before" and "after" DIR readings. To date, more than 80 percent of men who have tried the Six-Week Program noted a 20 percent improvement in their hardness numbers. This represents significant enhancement. More important, the long-term program put men on track not only to preserve sexual function, but also to actually begin to reverse underlying medical problems influencing hardness and health.

As I gained more knowledge about sexual medicine and experience with DIR, I also gained the confidence that I could help all of the men who came to see me. All men have the same doubts, the same concerns, and I can help with these problems.

> **B***ig Disappointment*
>
> For those men seeking penile enlargement surgery, the average gain in size is about one inch when flaccid and half an inch when erect. More than 65 percent of men who opt for penile enlargement surgery are dissatisfied with the results.

BEGINNING THE HARDNESS FACTOR PROGRAM

Every day each one of us, whether in his 20s, 30s, or even older than 60, is one day closer to ED, unless he is ready to make some positive changes in the way that he lives his life. I always explain to my younger patients that although their erections may be reliably hard now—1,500–2,000 grams of pressure on the DIR—they may have problems by the time they reach middle age. It is never too late or too early to start following my preventive program.

Dietary changes, regular exercise, and a variety of supplements that I will describe in the upcoming chapters can bring dramatic results in a man's hardness and overall sexual satisfaction. For more serious problems, pharmaceutical researchers have already found a way to naturally restore hardness with powerful prescription medications. But more important, these erection experts and I are in agreement that preventing the loss of erections will always be easier than restoring them. I am going to show you how. The sooner you rise to the challenge of taking care of your health and hardness, the sooner we can intervene in the battle and, with luck, do so while hardness problems are minimal or even imperceptible.

My patients understand this. They want to keep what they have attained. Keenly aware that they are at the peak of their lives, they want the new tools that will not only keep them mentally and physically fit, but actually better than someone years younger. In the realm of male sexuality, men can achieve this with the Hardness Factor.

As a doctor and a sexual medicine scientist, I know that the Hardness Factor will aid men in their 20s through their 70s and beyond, not only with their health and sexuality but in the sheer enjoyment of life.

My Ten Promises to You

1. If you are happy with your hardness now, you'll be even more pleased in as little as four days.

2. You can retain optimal hardness, sexual performance, and pleasure indefinitely.

3. You will heighten the sensitivity of your penis and have richer orgasms.

4. You will feel in peak condition all the time.

5. You will look and feel younger.

6. You'll jump-start energy systems.

7. You will recapture and improve physical strength and endurance.

8. You are going to protect and defend the body's most vital organs—the heart and brain.

9. You will maintain and improve the conditioning of the body, restoring a new, inner self-confidence.

10. You'll enhance the performance and sexual satisfaction of your partner.

► *THE STORY CONTINUES*

BILL, six weeks later

I was positive that after following the Hardness Factor Six-Week Program, Bill would have a new confidence in the bedroom. I hadn't asked him to deprive himself of anything in his life. I didn't ask him to start training for a marathon or switch to a macrobiotic diet. Instead, I wanted him to add positive behaviors and strengthen the many good health habits he already had. While I promised him that the program wouldn't be difficult to follow, I did promise that he would become much harder.

Six weeks after he walked into my office in a state of panic, Bill came for a follow-up visit. He was smiling—beaming, actually—and happy and said that he just couldn't have imagined the difference that six weeks could make in his sex life, his confidence, and surprisingly, in his relationship with Karen. He seemed enormously relieved.

I was glad to see that Bill's outlook had turned more positive. He admitted to initially doubting that a few simple changes in his diet and some supplements could make such a difference, but he was now a believer. "By the first week of the program, I knew something different was going on," he told me. "I woke up one day with a hard, morning erection—something I haven't had in a long time. By the next week, I felt a little firmer through my midsection, and a bit more flexible. By the fourth week, I was constantly looking at my calendar, counting the days to Karen's arrival. I not only wanted her, but really believed that I could please her," he said, laughing at himself. "When I finally picked her up at the airport and gave her a big kiss, I knew that I was no longer the same guy she had last been with in Santa Barbara."

Thanks to the Hardness Factor Six-Week Program, Bill now knows that he can get and enjoy an erection without concern. The softness, the self-doubts, the confusion, the anguish—they are no longer a part of his life. Bill clearly exuded a sense of contentment that I suspected he had not felt for quite some time. With the exception of venturing outside to take in a movie, he told me that he and Karen barely left the apartment the entire time she was in town. The lovemaking had been great, Bill admitted. "She tells me that it makes her feel great when she sees how much I want her."

I told Bill that his adherence to the program had produced the desired changes I knew were possible, but I also knew that if he continued with the program, the results would be even more significant. Not only would he be helping to preserve his sexual function as he got older, but he would actually begin to reverse any underlying medical problems that could affect his hardness and health.

GOOD HARD LESSONS

Lesson 1 Hardness issues affect young men and are of great concern.

Lesson 2 Having hardness problems does not mean that you have erectile dysfunction and need the aid of prescription drugs.

Lesson 3 Lifestyle changes will not only change but positively affect the hardness of a man's penis.

Lesson 4 Knowledge is power. Understanding the secret of increasing the strength of your hardness can ultimately change the nature of your erections. Success breeds more success (and pleasure and smiles).

ON SEXUAL MEDICINE—MENTAL, EMOTIONAL, AND PHYSICAL

The Hardness Factor is a medical book focusing on important physical issues that affect male sexuality. Unfortunately, biologic concerns (about hardness issues especially) often act as effective barriers to romance and intimacy. My aim is to help men overcome these various hurdles so they can reclaim their sex lives.

It is certainly understood that great, satisfying sex is more than a hard penis and that there are many emotional and psychological aspects that help build strong, loving, and deeply satisfying relationships between partners. For those people searching for answers concerning love and intimacy, many wonderful books effectively cover these topics. However, *The Hardness Factor* is strictly a book about sexual medicine and I am only going to deal with those concerns specific to men.

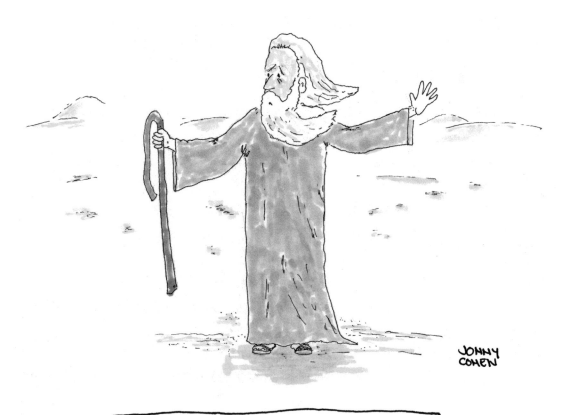

MOSES, THE MID-LIFE YEARS

66 *Welcome to my submarine lair. It's long, hard, and full of seamen.*

Dr. Evil,
Goldmember

2

A HARD MAN IS GOOD TO FIND

ERECTIONS COME FROM THE HEART >>>

Men are by their very nature hard. Strength, self-confidence, and determination are all good, powerful male attributes. The hardness of a man's erection is the window to his overall health, self-confidence, and contentment. When hardness waivers, it is often the earliest sign of compromised health and a diminution of quality of life. My goal is to help men maintain maximum hardness for life.

Heart Health = Hard and Healthy

ARCHIE, age 42—a wife's concern

Rebecca was in my office without her husband's knowledge. Worried and extremely upset, the 36-year-old college history professor had come to talk to me about her husband, Archie, and his recent lack of hardness. This was something he had originally made light of, and now refused even to acknowledge. While Rebecca admitted sex used to be regular and exciting for the couple, she and Archie had not had relations for the past seven weeks. This estrangement was of particular concern to her because their relationship had always been close. The lack of sex was now driving a powerful wedge between them.

I knew Archie's father very well. I had treated Big Archie for years, right up until his death a few months earlier from heart failure. He was only 70. Unfortunately, Archie was following his father's example. His pack-a-day smoking habit, developed as a teen, a clear family history of heart disease, his long-time struggles with his weight, and now his failing erections at age 42 were clear harbingers of underlying atherosclerosis, the fatty deposits that begin to narrow the arteries and cause a host of health issues. This is exactly what I explained to Rebecca.

"There is no such thing as a sudden heart attack," I told her. "It is something that people develop day by day, over the years, after accumulating a lifetime of unhealthy habits. While he certainly does not know it, Archie's heart status is linked directly to the performance of his penis. When atherosclerosis starts to develop, it begins to clog up the tiny vessels in the penis. The impact is often seen there first, long before it ever shows up in the coronary arteries of the heart, or in any of the other 100,000 miles of blood vessels in the body.

"When blood flow is slowed down to the penis due to the gunking up of these tiny penile arteries—they're only as wide as the dot atop the letter *i*—hardness is diminished as the plasticity, the suppleness of the blood vessels, is compromised. This leaves the blood vessels less responsive and stiff. Allowed to progress without any therapy, the blood vessel walls thicken, and the lumen—the space inside the vessel—becomes smaller. Blood flow is restricted even more and erections lose their hardness."

Problems getting or keeping an erection are all too often a red flag, a marker for heart trouble now or sometime in the near future. I figured that Archie had some underlying heart disease that trig-

*S*moke More, Get Less

According to a study at the University of Kentucky, men who were nonsmokers reported having sex twelve times a month, whereas those who smoked had sex only six times.

gered his hardness problems, but he was just too embarrassed to talk about it or take any proactive steps to reverse it. "If he doesn't seek help, very soon he could end up like Big Archie," I told Rebecca.

I wanted to help both Archie and Rebecca. Since Archie, like so many men, was reluctant to see a doctor unless he was carried there by ambulance, I encouraged her to get him in to see me as soon as possible under the pretense that it was time for his annual flu shot. I assured her I would do my best to help restore his heart health, which would enhance his hardness at the same time. By following my Hardness Factor Six-Week Program, Archie's health and hardness would hopefully experience a quick turnaround.

As the plasticity returned to his blood vessels by following my recommendations for nutrition, supplements, and exercise over the next forty-two days, he would produce more of an important molecule called nitric oxide, or NO. With increased NO levels, he would see a significant impact in the health of his blood vessels and his hardness.

ALL IN THE FAMILY LESSONS

Lesson 1　Atherosclerosis starts its deadly course many years in advance of symptoms.

Lesson 2　Diminished hardness should be acknowledged as an early warning of heart disease, especially when it occurs in a younger man.

Lesson 3　Don't play the denial game—tell your doctor about your concerns. Men can experience quick turnarounds in hardness and health when atherosclerosis is caught in the early stages.

HARDNESS IS AN EARLY WARNING INDICATOR

Men are sometimes taken aback when I start talking to them about their heart when they have come to see me about their penis. Others are equally surprised when I bring up hardness issues when they have come to see me about their heart. They soon find out, however, that the links between the two are powerful, as are the common risk factors that negatively influence each. These include the following:

▶ High cholesterol, especially LDL-C
(low-density lipoprotein cholesterol)
▶ Hypertension
▶ Depression and stress
▶ Smoking
▶ Weight

The performances of the penis and the heart are linked together for life. The more men begin to understand the importance of maintaining hardness, the more they will understand about maintaining a healthy heart. And the more they come to understand about the heart, the more they will come to appreciate what the Hardness Factor Six-Week Program has to offer in terms of establishing and sustaining optimal health for life.

Like the canary in the coal mine warning of unseen danger, men need to be aware that the health of their penis—more specifically, the hardness of their erections—is a great early-warning indicator of any underlying cardiovascular problems that may be developing. I tell all my patients that if they are serious about preventing hardness and heart problems, they need to start fighting the degeneration that is brought on by lifestyle factors, and take the steps necessary to achieve the optimal health of both the penis and the heart.

> ## Your Heart, Mind, and Penis
>
> Taking care of your hardness positively impacts your heart health. Scientists are now reporting that it may also play a major role in warding off Alzheimer's disease (AD) as well. At the International Conference on Alzheimer's in 2004, researchers reported that there was a major relationship between good heart health and a lower risk of Alzheimer's, the mind-robbing disease that now afflicts more than 4.5 million Americans. This comes about by raising good cholesterol (HDL-C) through regular exercise and proper nutrition, lowering blood pressure, and preventing diabetes. I will take this positive message a step further: When you take care of your hardness, you will be taking care of the health of not only your penis and heart, but your mind as well.

PUTTING THE PENIS ON THE COUCH

In the early twentieth century, a major theme emerged in the nascent field of sexual medicine. Sigmund Freud emphasized the contribution of psychogenic factors—oftentimes disturbing childhood experiences that led to erection difficulties. With a psychiatrist's help, Freud felt, the patient would acknowledge these traumatic episodes from the past in the hope that their recognition would then lead to the resolution of any hardness problems.

Unfortunately, this process was long, arduous, and often worthless, as the man on the doctor's couch still suffered from weak or infrequent erections. Freud's powerful psychiatric concepts—which influenced both the definition of male erection problems and its treatment—were regarded as dogma in many parts of the world until the 1980s. With the advent of Viagra in the 1990s, his concepts on erection problems became essentially nothing but sexual medicine footnotes.

While there are many men who do have serious psychological components to their erection difficulties, it is now well understood that in almost every case there is also a powerful physiological root to their hardness problem. The psychological component is often a response to their erection difficulties, manifested as depression or anxiety. Rarely are psychological problems the sole cause of hardness difficulties.

ELIMINATING THE SEXUAL CONFIDENCE GAP

With Freud's theories about erectile dysfunction now largely discredited, let me state that when it comes to sexual performance with men, it often boils down to issues of confidence. Thanks to my early work with prescription erection drugs, I saw firsthand that most men with advanced erectile dysfunction had no sexual confidence whatsoever. They had lost it all, even the younger men, as the erection failures started to accumulate. Becoming intimate with a partner was an invitation to embarrassment and shame. What I didn't realize, however, was that many men without severe erection problems, some in their mid- to late 20s, already had burgeoning concerns about their sexual confidence.

> *L*ong Live the King!
>
> The condom is said to be named for the Earl of Condom, a British physician at the court of Charles II who was asked by the king to design something to keep him from developing syphilis. The oiled sheep intestine was a big hit, and it was soon used by noblemen and commoners alike.

My preliminary research with the Digital Inflection Rigidometer revealed that, at times, a good percentage of young, seemingly healthy men have difficulty obtaining and maintaining a firm erection. This points out fairly graphically that there is a *sexual confidence gap* among men 20 and older that is silent, not discussed or shared among friends or physicians.

Over the years, many of these men eventually opened up to me, complaining that there was often an inordinate delay between the onset of sexual stimulation to peak erectile hardness. That delay was very disconcerting. Add a condom to the mix and erections were often lost for that intimate lovemaking session.

In addition, once the man started worrying about his erections, it snowballed, leading to less-than-satisfactory erections in his next encounters. All it takes for a man is one failure with a partner, one mind-body disconnect, and anxiety will set in. If allowed to continue without any intervention, relationships can quickly become strained.

WHAT IS YOUR HARDNESS RISK?

Understanding that there is a very strong link between hardness and heart health, I want you to figure out your current risk for developing heart disease and hardness problems over the next decade. You will first need to know your full lipid profile and systolic blood pressure (the first number). Yes, you will need to pick up the phone—call your doctor and make an appointment. A simple blood test and blood pressure exam given by your doctor will supply you with these numbers. The blood test will measure the following:

▶ Total cholesterol, the combination of LDL-C and HDL-C

▶ Low-density lipoprotein (LDL or "bad") cholesterol

▶ High-density lipoprotein (HDL or "good") cholesterol

The National Cholesterol Education Program has developed a point and percentage system that I have adapted to help you determine your risk of hardness problems and potential heart attack. There are five categories to assess—so let's get started.

*P*revu: New Skin Test
for Heart Disease

Prevu is a new in-office, three-minute test that measures cholesterol in the palm of your hand, helping detect heart disease without drawing a blood sample. After placing a thin foam pad on the palm, the doctor puts a special liquid enzyme onto the pad, which soon causes a color change depending on the amount of cholesterol in the skin. A hand-held device measures the color change and correlates cholesterol level.

To determine your risk in each of the five categories, circle the number that best describes your situation.

LEGEND

Category 1	
HEART/HARDNESS FACTOR RISK ASSESSMENT	
Risk Factor	**Risk Point**
AGE	
Less than 34	-1
35–39	0
40–44	1
45–49	2
50–54	3
55–59	4
60–64	5
65–69	6
70–74	7

* This formula is also found at HTTP://HIN.NHLBI.NIH.GOV/ATPIII/CALCULATOR.ASP

Category 2	
HEART/HARDNESS FACTOR RISK ASSESSMENT	
Risk Factor	**Risk Point**
TOTAL CHOLESTEROL (mg/dL)	
Less than 160	-3
160–199	0
200–239	1
240–279	2
Greater than 280	3

TOTAL CHOLESTEROL > Total cholesterol is the sum of all the cholesterol in your blood. The higher your total cholesterol, the greater your risk for heart disease and hardness problems. Here are the total values that matter:

Less than 160 mg/dL > "Desirable" level that puts you at a very low risk for heart disease and hardness problems.

160–199 mg/dL > "High" level. There may be some hardness problems.

200 mg/dL and above > "Very high" blood cholesterol. You have more than twice the risk of heart disease compared to someone whose cholesterol is below 200 mg/dL. You can expect many hardness problems.

LDL CHOLESTEROL > LDL-C levels are used to determine your risk of developing heart and hardness problems. These are the LDL-C values I recommend for my patients:

LDL-C less than 100 mg/dL > if you have heart disease or diabetes. While not yet proven, I believe in the near future that the next goal for everyone will be to achieve this level. I currently urge all of my patients to aim for this.

LDL-C less than 130 mg/dL > if you have two or more risk factors.*

* Risk factors include cigarette smoking, hypertension, low HDL (less than 40 mg/dL), family history of heart disease, age (55 or older), being overweight, and failure to exercise regularly.

HDL CHOLESTEROL > (HDL-C) is the so-called good cholesterol. HDL-C carries cholesterol in the blood from other parts of the body back to the liver, which leads to its removal from the body. HDL-C helps keep cholesterol from building up in the walls of the arteries and forming dangerous plaques.

Here are the vital HDL-C levels that matter:

Less than 35 mg/dL > A major risk factor for heart disease and hardness problems.

35–59 mg/dL > In the good range.

60 mg/dL and above > Highly protective against heart disease. Hardness levels should be extremely high.

Category 3

HEART/HARDNESS FACTOR RISK ASSESSMENT

Risk Factor	Risk Point
HDL CHOLESTEROL (mg/dL)	
Less than 35	2
35–44	1
45–49	0
50–59	0
Greater than 60	–2

SYSTOLIC BLOOD PRESSURE > Systolic blood pressure is the first number of your blood pressure reading. For example, if your reading is 120/80 (120 over 80), your systolic blood pressure is 120.

Category 4

HEART/HARDNESS FACTOR RISK ASSESSMENT

Risk Factor	Risk Point
SYSTOLIC BLOOD PRESSURE (mmHg)	
Less than 120	0
120–129	0
130–139	1
140–159	2
160	3

SMOKER > Select "yes" if you have smoked any cigarettes in the past month. Smoking constricts blood vessels and affects hardness.

Category 5

HEART/HARDNESS FACTOR RISK ASSESSMENT

Risk Factor	Risk Point
SMOKER	
No	0
Yes	2

NOTE: If you smoke more than one pack per day, add another point.

ADDITIONAL POINTS

○ If you already have a family history of heart disease, add two points.

○ If you are a regular exerciser and work out at least five times a week, subtract one point.

○ If you exercise three times or less per week, add one point.

○ If you are overweight or obese, add one point.

TOTAL UP YOUR POINTS FROM THE CATEGORIES ABOVE

Age + Total Cholesterol + HDL-C + Systolic + Smoker = _____

TOTAL POINTS _____

WHAT YOUR SCORE MEANS

○ **3 points or less:** You are in good heart health and your hardness is exceptional.

○ **4–6 points:** You are at moderate risk for developing heart disease and you probably have already had some hardness failures.

○ **7–10 points:** You are at high risk for heart disease and a heart attack during the next ten years. Your hardness level is probably low and you have probably experienced many erectile problems already.

○ **More than 10 points:** You are at very high risk for heart disease and heart attack and have advanced atherosclerosis that is dangerously clogging your arteries. Your hardness level is extremely low or nonexistent.

A little sobering? If you are like the majority of men, you have the usual denial mechanisms and comfortable "it's never going to happen to me" syndrome. Heart and hardness problems are a fact of life—your life. But you can do something about them—and we will, together.

YOUR RISK OF HEART ATTACK/STROKE/HARDNESS PROBLEMS IN THE NEXT DECADE	
Points	Your Risk (%)
0	2
1	3
2	4
3	5
4	7
5	8
6	10
7	13
8	16
9	20
10	25
11	31
12	37
13	45
14	50+
15	50+

Now, using your final point total, locate your number of total points on the list. This will indicate your ten-year risk of having a heart attack and hardness problems, expressed as a percentage.

My 10–year risk is_____

HARDNESS 101

Before going any further with our understanding of hardness, it helps to understand how erections occur in the first place. An erection is actually dependent upon the finely orchestrated actions of muscles, nerves, and blood vessels in the penis. Additionally, it requires good blood flow, which is regulated by the nervous system, to bring about the hydraulic or lifting action. The change in the penis from flaccid (soft) to tumescent (swollen) to erect (hard) is caused by an intricate partnership involving the brain, blood vessels, nerves, and hormones.

The natural state of the penis is flaccid. An erection begins when the brain senses something arousing: a beautiful person in a bathing suit, an erotic image, a whispered inducement. This is your libido at work and it is the first step in taking your penis from its limp, flaccid state to maximum hardness.

Impulses are then fired off from the brain to the lower part of the back, through the pelvis, and then to the penis. Nerve stimulation, induced by messages sent by nitric oxide, causes the smooth muscles of the penis to relax. This allows increased quantities of blood to flow in through the right and left cavernosal arteries, filling the space within the cavernosa. For the blood to fill the penis and cause it to become longer, wider, and harder, it has to multiply to about six times its normal flow. Like a sponge, the corpora tissues quickly expand with blood, engorging and enlarging the penis. **(See Appendix V, page 329.)**

Then, as the corpora cavernosa continue to swell like two oversized water balloons, they finally press against the veins that normally allow blood to flow out, effectively preventing it from leaving. Finally, packed with blood, the corpora become rigid and erect, making the penis hard enough for penetration. **The more blood that flows in, the longer this inflow is maintained, and the longer the outflow is prevented, the longer an erection will be sustained.**

*P*ut *That Away!*

Though nudity was acceptable, an exposed erection was frowned upon in ancient Greece.

*A*tta' *Boy!*

The male fetus is capable of attaining an erection during the last trimester of pregnancy.

THE REFRACTORY PERIOD—COME AGAIN?

Once an orgasm occurs—or a man becomes distracted, disinterested, or distressed—the erection begins its process of detumescence. As this occurs, the penile veins open, blood drains out, and the penis becomes flaccid once again.

The refractory period is the temporary recovery period between ejaculations in which a man cannot be sexually aroused to further orgasm. This may be the result of a temporary rise in a hormone called prolactin. A drug is currently in development to reduce the refractory period. (Is this a great time to be a man, or what?)

When is it possible to reload and be ready for another orgasm? Several critical factors come into play:

▶ **Your Hardness Factor.** Underlying risk factors will cause a delay.

▶ **Age.** Youth (and good health) is in your favor. In your 20s, a second hard erection and orgasm is possible within minutes. Thirty to forty years later, decreases in nerve function and underlying atherosclerosis may stretch the refractory period to a day.

▶ **Libido.** A healthy appetite for sex, regular sexual activity, and a willing partner play important roles in triggering follow-up erections and orgasm.

> **N**ot Including Wilt Chamberlain
>
> The average number of times a healthy male will ejaculate in a lifetime is 7,200. Of this number, approximately 2,000 times will result from masturbation.

A HARD NIGHT'S SLEEP

Hard erections depend on regular and vast supplies of oxygen-rich blood. If a man goes without an erection for an extended period, he could be setting himself up for a major hardness setback. By depriving the penile cells of oxygen, over time the muscle cells begin to lose their natural elasticity and become replaced by scar tissue. This tissue is less elastic and limits hardness when you finally do achieve an erection.

Nonetheless, the body still tries to take care of itself and regularly primes its own pump. Unknown to most, men have the most powerful erections of their lives while they are in the rapid eye movement (REM) portion of nighttime sleep. During this deep dream state, a man can have anywhere from three to five spontaneous erections in this six- to eight-hour sleep span. Blood engorges the penis, bringing it to full attention, oftentimes for an hour or longer. These powerful erections have nothing to do with sexual dreams, however. Researchers now believe these nocturnal occurrences are nature's way of protecting and preserving the elastic penile tissues within the corpora cavernosa. Yes, Mother Nature likes her men hard.

THE DA VINCI MODE

Of all the people who helped launch the Renaissance, none was more remarkable than Leonardo da Vinci. Granted, there were some who may have equaled him as an artist, but there was no greater scientific visionary when it came to drawing the intricate parts of the human body. Da Vinci's anatomical studies, drawn from cadavers at the local morgue, were used not only to aid him in his understanding of anatomy, but also as a means to understand how the body worked and moved.

> 66 The penis does not obey the order of its master, who tries to erect or shrink it at will, whereas instead the penis erects freely while its master is asleep. The penis must be said to have its own mind.
>
> LEONARDO DA VINCI

Among his other achievements, da Vinci, who died in 1519, was one of the first—and most adept—at creating anatomically correct medical drawings of the human penis. Shortly after he was given access to the local hospital morgue in Florence, he began to fill his notebooks with drawings of the internal workings of the penis.

After lengthy visits to the hospital, da Vinci came to understand that blood filled the erect penis—not air, as had previously been thought. This discovery, which he noted in his sketchbooks, came one hundred years before the official pronouncement by the great Ambroise Paré, the French physician, who is now recognized as the "father of modern surgery."

However, what neither da Vinci nor Paré could have understood at the time was that while blood does in fact fill the erect penis, that is not what creates the erection. The erection and the strength of its hardness factor depend almost exclusively on the amount of nitric oxide (NO) in the penis. And when something goes wrong with nitric oxide production, hardness is adversely affected.

A NOBEL PRIZE–WINNING PENIS

Nitric oxide comes from the conjoining of our atmosphere's two most abundant gases, nitrogen and oxygen. Surprisingly, though, there is now ample evidence that NO is one of the most important and versatile chemical messengers in the entire body—especially in the penis.

The erection of the penis during sexual excitation is due in great part to the NO released from nerve endings close to the blood vessels of the penis and from NO made on the endothelium, the inner lining of the blood vessels. Relaxation of these vessels causes blood to pool in the blood sinuses, resulting in a hard erection suitable for penetration. The healthier a man is, the more NO he produces, the harder the erection.

Nitric oxide is not only important in the cardiovascular system, but in the central nervous system, the brain. NO fights infection and inflammation. It is also important in the gastrointestinal tract, helping to prevent ulcers and stimulating the movement of food throughout the tract. It also aids air flow in lungs and controls bladder and erectile function. NO is such a widespread signaling molecule within the body that when its multitude of actions was finally uncovered, the researchers were awarded a Nobel Prize in 1998.

SAYING YES TO NO

Now that you understand why NO is important, you will understand the value of increasing NO production in the body. In the Hardness Factor Six-Week Program I recommend regular exercise, plus a supplement that will improve blood flow, lower blood pressure, and protect against coronary heart disease and plaque formation. What we have learned over the last few years is that the body's most potent way of stimulating NO formation in endothelial cells is exercise. Even mild exercise, such as walking. The reason is simple. When you exercise, blood flow increases; it rushes through the arteries faster.

When that blood rushes through the endothelial cells, it turns them on to make more NO. That is why exercise is good for your health. In order for NO to be effective, it has to be produced continuously.

So how can we keep up NO production? First, by saying "no" to smoking, fatty foods, and that sedentary lifestyle. Increasing L-arginine consumption is one way to increase NO presence because the arginine in food is converted to nitric oxide in the body. This important amino acid, a building block of proteins, is found in meat, cereals, fish, nuts, milk, and certain vegetables.

Since most people do not get enough arginine from their diet, I want men to take an L-arginine supplement. I will explain more about this in Chapter Four.

Antioxidants, like vitamins E and C, also work to protect NO against destruction from oxidative stress—helping maintain NO production. You find these antioxidants in Pycnogenol, marine fish oils, and other supplements that I recommend in my Six-Week Program. Each is a potent fighter of free radicals, the molecules that damage NO in the endothelium. When you take them together, you will be assured of maximum NO production, complete heart protection, and ultimate hardness.

Sex and the Heart (Attack)

CHARLIE, age 40—Basic training

Charlie was scared. The 40-year-old artist was describing the account of a well-known local politician who had suffered a fatal heart attack while having sex. "Dying while in the saddle is a nice way to go," he admitted, "but I was wondering how one can avoid the heart attack part. I happen to find death during sex to be a bit disconcerting."

While rare, suffering a lethal heart attack during sex is certainly not unique. According to research published in *The Journal of the American Medical Association,* a man's risk of suffering a lethal heart attack increases during the two hours after having sex.

"What about the guy like me, who isn't in the greatest shape? What is my risk?" Charlie wanted to know.

"Sex is a physical act," I said, "and every physical act is associated with an increased risk for heart problems for a short period after the act is completed, whether it be swimming, running, or sex.

"From beginning to end, according to researchers, the amount of physical activity during sex is about the same as you would get in walking up two flights of stairs, or playing a 21-point game of table tennis. However, one man's romp is another man's nap. Since sex is a physical act, your risk of suffering a heart attack is about 2.5 chances in a million. Any man who is in good shape, with no heart disease, should have little fear of inducing a heart attack while having sex."

I then posed a scenario to Charlie that I had already posed to countless other patients who wanted to know why they needed to be in good shape for sex. "Here's the deal. It's Monday night," I said. "On Friday night I want you to be timed for running the 100-meter dash. Over the next four days, I want you to prepare by stretching, lifting weights, eating properly, and training on the track. Come Friday, I am going to take out my stopwatch and time you.

> 66 Sex is like an athletic event and takes careful planning if you are going to turn in your best result.

"On the night of your race against the clock, you are going to have a very light meal and then go to the track. If everything goes well, you will turn in a very good time for yourself."

Charlie wanted to know what running 100 meters had to do with sex.

"Everything," I said. "Sex is like an athletic event and takes careful planning if you are going to turn in your best result. You want to be in great shape so you are ready for your 100-meter workout in the bedroom. This entails eating sensibly, limiting alcohol, not smoking, and getting enough sleep. When the gun goes off, you will be primed and ready."

I handed Charlie a photocopy of my Hardness Factor Six-Week Program. "You will be a different man, in and out of the bedroom, when you finish this," I said. "And you won't be worrying about a heart attack anymore. I can assure you of that."

SEXUAL FITNESS LESSONS

Lesson 1 Passionate sex requires higher levels of physical fitness.

Lesson 2 Sex is a form of physical exertion that can be harmful to men with advanced heart disease if they are not in shape for the activity.

Lesson 3 In a study of healthy married men ages 25 to 43, foreplay took three to six minutes, while orgasm lasted an average of ten to sixteen seconds.

Lesson 4 The highest heart rate in the above study, which was recorded with the man-on-top position, was 127 beats per minute. This was 67 percent of the maximum heart rate, a relatively high rate for the nonathletic.

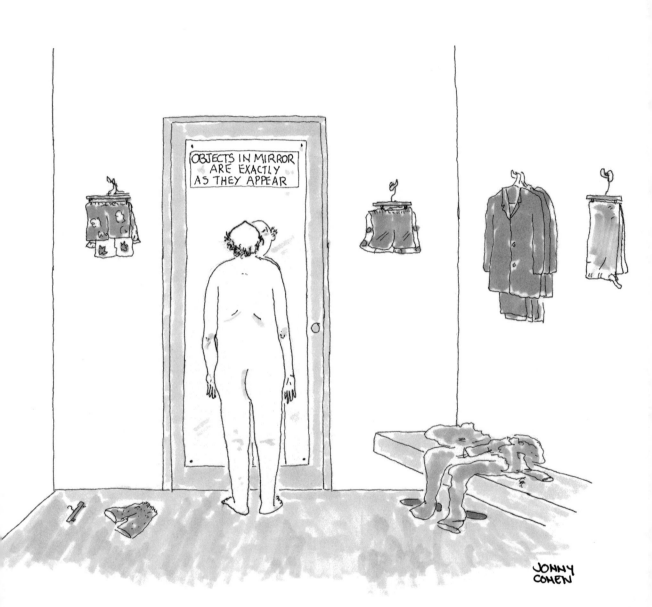

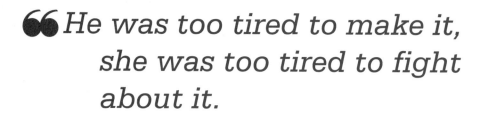

" *He was too tired to make it, she was too tired to fight about it.*

"Life in the Fast Lane,"
The Eagles

3

THE HARDNESS FACTOR SIX-WEEK PROGRAM

BETTER HEALTH, BETTER SEX, BETTER LIFE >>>>>>>>>>>>>>>>>>>>>>

The Hardness Factor Six-Week Program is a rejuvenating health therapy that is also the best non-pharmacological hardness regimen. Men will often blame their bouts of "softness" on getting older, bad luck, fate, or poor genes, but staying hard is actually a lifestyle decision that you make. In the next six chapters, I will provide all the key components to ensure that you achieve results. Hard is good; harder is better.

Hardness in Both Body and Mind

RON, age 41—Where did Buster go?

I had a new patient sitting in front of me who said he wanted to talk about a "personal problem." I knew from past experience with patients that personal problems could range from wanting to find out how to prevent hair loss to what to do about postnasal drip.

It turned out that Ron was a prime example of the "new" patient I am now treating, all thanks to Viagra and the other erection drugs. Ron was 41, an ad executive with a successful career, and he had plenty of dates every night of the week. "A friend at work said you had given him some vitamins especially formulated for the penis and he's very happy with them," he said. "I'd like some of them, too. I'm concerned about my sex life."

I asked Ron what he meant.

"I have to find a way so that when I go out on a date, I can be assured, 100 percent assured, that when it comes time to go to bed, I won't be thinking that I may not be able to perform. I don't want the thought anywhere in my mind. That's what I mean."

Ron was handsome, soft-spoken, introspective, and clearly frustrated. He admitted that he was in a rut, no, make that a hole. A deep, dark hole. Although he had plenty of female companionship, he admitted he found it difficult to go out on dates because of his overriding lack of sexual confidence. This low self-confidence, he felt, was directly caused by his inability to maintain a consistently strong erection.

"Whenever I am with a woman, I'm never sure if I'll be able to get hard and keep it hard," he said.

I knew I could help Ron, but first I needed some more information. I asked him if he could regularly get an erection.

"Sure," he said. "When I have sex, it just isn't consistently hard all the way through. I worry that it's going to disappear during sex."

"Has it disappeared before?" I asked.

"In college I never had a problem. Losing an erection never crossed my mind. Now I think about Buster all the time. Buster is not working like he used to. It started about a year ago. As I'm kissing a woman and starting to become intimate, I start to feel he is going somewhere else. Although I'm kissing a woman and touching her, at the same time, I'm worried what Buster is doing."

"Buster. Is that your name for your penis?"

But Will You Serve Hard Time?

In 2000, the Mississippi state legislature introduced a bill to make it illegal for a man to have an erection at a strip club even if he is fully dressed.

Ron was clearly embarrassed now. "Yeah, it's Buster. I call it Buster."

"Giving a name to your penis is a form of dislocation and it's common with men," I explained to Ron. "What you really need to do is claim your penis and establish your ownership. Until you do that, you don't own it and your hardness problems will persist because you are separating yourself from your body and who you are. You have to take responsibility for your penis, just as you do everything else in your life. Claim it. Own it. Enjoy it. Until your penis is part of the man named Ron, your hardness problems will continue.

"You need to figure out who you are and what is going wrong," I said. "If you have a sprained ankle, you don't say, '*Jim* got hurt.' And you don't consider yourself less of a man because you sprain your ankle. It's the same when you have problems with your penis. You have a medical problem, Ron. Something is physiologically wrong with you and it's affecting your hardness.

"However, the good news is that there are definitely solutions. Just as you have trained yourself for failure, I am going to give you a plan to follow that will restore your hardness and help you reclaim your sexual confidence. I am going to retrain you so you are in the best sexual shape of your life."

As I explained to Ron, hardness is something all men can have, and in most cases, they won't have to rely on Cialis, Levitra, or Viagra. There is a better way to hardness and health. Following the Hardness Factor Six-Week Program was a great start. I outlined some suggestions for him, each guaranteed to bolster maximum hardness.

It all starts by having the responsibility to be accountable for yourself. When we are healthy and hard, our quality of life is good. I told Ron that taking care of his body and losing the extra twenty pounds he was carrying was the first step in his recovery process. The excess weight he had put on during the past two years of expense-account dinners, coupled with no exercise and a tendency to drink too much, had significantly affected his ability to get a hard erection. Smoking cigars added to the problem. Pulling all-nighters to finish projects didn't help either.

I told Ron that taking better care of himself was the first positive step to getting on with his life. I wanted him to get in shape for sex, eating judiciously to enhance hardness and taking a variety of prosexual supplements that would prime his system for maximum hardness.

It sounded a little radical: enhanced hardness and sexual confidence in a little more than a month, without any erection drugs. As Ron sat there, I could tell that a light had suddenly clicked on. He now understood. He wanted desperately to turn his life around and he was willing to try the program to help make these important lifestyle changes.

DATING LESSONS

Lesson 1 Understand that your penis is an integral part of your physical self.

Lesson 2 If your perceived hardness level changes, there is often a physical—and reversible—cause.

Lesson 3 As great as the success and importance of the new sexual medicine is, it is important to enjoy and strengthen what you have, naturally.

HARD IS GOOD; HARDER IS BETTER

In addition to significantly enhancing your health, the Hardness Factor Six-Week Program will help you develop more penile hardness than ever before. Your erections will become stronger. You will stay harder longer. In just six weeks, you will significantly enhance your bedroom abilities. Fatigue will be banished and your stamina, strength, and flexibility boosted, giving you added energy and vitality. You will make steady and significant gains in how you feel, beginning with your very first day. These gains will accumulate and in just six weeks, you will:

Improve heart function. A strong heart can pump more blood through the body with every beat. Like the other muscles, the heart becomes stronger through regular physical activity, specific supplements, and smart eating. A fit heart will also pump more blood at this maximum level and can sustain it longer with less strain. Recent studies have reported that the "elasticity" of the heart, which is created through regular physical activity, is critical to maintaining a healthy cardiovascular system.

Improve cholesterol levels. Cholesterol, the waxy substance found in the bloodstream, helps form cell membranes, some hormones, and a variety of tissues. My eating, supplement, and exercise suggestions have the ability to boost protective HDL (the "good" cholesterol) levels, while lowering LDL ("bad" cholesterol) blood levels. Remember: a high HDL level, defined as 45 mg/dL or more, is considered to be extremely protective against coronary heart disease—and hardness problems.

Prevent or combat obesity. Most men not only eat too much, but they also eat too much of the wrong foods—fast food, fried food, sweets, and "empty calories" with no nutritional value. To top it off, we are not as physically active as we should be during the day. Therefore, it comes as no surprise that we have become a nation of fat people. Almost 35 percent of Americans are now considered obese. And that's not the end of it.

Obesity is a primary risk factor for heart disease and is linked to many other ailments as well, including diabetes, high cholesterol, high blood pressure, certain cancers, gallstones, and degenerative arthritis. You can add erectile dysfunction to this list.

The Hardness Factor Six-Week Program will lead to effective and permanent weight loss. Even small weight losses are associated with a

> **I**t's a Good Thing
>
> Nothing can lift a man's spirits more than an effortless erection. Think what a happy thought that is—now wipe that smile off your face.

decrease in cardiovascular risk, improved hardness, better glucose tolerance, lower blood pressure, and an enhanced cholesterol profile. Who knew that skipping *Super Size* could help you **SUPER SIZE**.

Boost self-esteem. The psychological catharsis you undergo during the next six weeks may match or surpass your physiologic changes. Feeling healthier and harder can raise your self-esteem, making you feel more confident, assertive, and attractive.

Boost sexual intimacy. Just as a hard erection is a barometer of a man's overall health, having regular sex is a barometer that indicates the overall health of a relationship. Sex, which includes intercourse and erotic touching, is an essential component to an intimate and healthy relationship.

MY HARDNESS PRESCRIPTION

The goal of the program is to make you stronger, more active, slimmer, mobile, energetic, vigorous, and confident. In a phrase: hard, healthy, and happy. Regardless of how old you are, how much you weigh, how strong you are, and your current personal status, just follow the program for six weeks and you will be creating a dynamic lifestyle of nutrition and exercise that will enhance your overall health and hardness. Sex will be better, too.

66 The choice to live better, longer, and harder is yours to make.

As you will soon see, the program is graduated and takes all levels of health and physical stamina into account—you progress according to your individual ability. And everyone—no matter what shape they are currently in—will experience increased hardness and sexual capability. The choice to live better, longer, and harder is yours to make. With the Hardness Factor Six-Week Program, I am offering you the ultimate hardness prescription. Now, it's up to you to fill it. Take charge of your life and make the commitment to hardness.

Not Worth the Weight

A recent two-year study in Italy of overweight and obese men reported a 30 percent chance of developing erectile dysfunction. This is not actually surprising, since approximately 8 out of 10 men with moderate to severe hardness problems tip the scales at much more than their ideal weight.

However, the Italian researchers wanted to find out if a simple lifestyle modification program of exercise and dietary changes could make a difference in the hardness of the extra-large men. The scientists enrolled men 35 to 55 years old who were obese and complained of hardness issues. They were then divided into two groups: one which included an exercise and nutrition program, and the other, which only instructed the members how to lose weight.

After twenty-four months, those men who exercised not only lost weight but also one-third of them had a restoration of hardness. The more weight lost, the better the hardness and overall satisfaction.

The reasons for the return of hardness with this drug-free approach are linked to a combination of factors revealed in the Hardness Factor Six-Week Program: increased nitric oxide production, healthier arteries, restoration of self-confidence, and enhanced sexual confidence.

THE HARDNESS FACTOR: AN OVERVIEW

The Hardness Factor Program has been designed to maximize results over a six-week span. All you have to do is follow my suggestions for each week and you are guaranteed to see and feel positive changes. My supplement recommendations will increase sexual interest and enhance the all-important nitric oxide production and endothelial health. At the end of six weeks, you will have succeeded in restoring your health and hardness, allowing you to lay total claim to the pleasure that you deserve in your sexual relationships.

The sexual fitness exercises I recommend are not difficult, nor do they require special equipment. They will work all the basic muscle groups, ensuring balanced strength and stable joints. I do want you to increase your daily physical activity, so I am going to ask you to walk. This will help pare away body fat as it increases optimal heart function.

SENSUOUS NUTRITION: A CONNECTION TO HARDNESS

More than 2,500 years ago, Hippocrates, the father of medicine, said, "Let food be your medicine and medicine be your food." It has taken some time for scientists to finally address this Hippocratic dictum, but we do know that people who consume plenty of vegetables, fruits, and grains and who exercise regularly are less likely to develop heart disease and hardness problems than those who do not.

Several years ago, I began to wonder if it was possible to use food, or some particular nutrient, as preventive medicine against hardness problems and subsequent heart disease. Of course, I realize that I am not alone with this idea. All over the world, scientists in many disciplines are studying diet as never before—for the first time, trying to understand exactly how specific foods work in the body, right down to which particular enzymes are helped or hurt by what we eat and drink.

The search for health answers in the supermarket is certainly not an easy assignment. People eat about two to three pounds of food each day. Trying to sort out which food or particular nutrient—or something that has been cooked in oil, baked, broiled, steamed, or raw—has a particular protective effect on a certain gene or organ is an extremely complicated and time-consuming scientific effort.

Even so, it seems increasingly obvious that, from a health standpoint, the rich Western diet—notoriously high in animal fats and poor in grains, fruits, and vegetables—leaves a lot to be desired, on many different levels.

Over the years, I have encountered many patients who took good care of their health, only to have their efforts undermined by what they choose to eat. My point is that making wise food choices is just as important to your success in the Hardness Factor Six-Week Program as exercising and taking your supplements. What you eat and when you eat it will go a long way to keeping you energetic, fueling your body, and priming it to build lean body tissue while paring away excess body fat. I want to address all of these concerns over the course of the next forty-two days.

When it comes to hardness and sex, I also believe that a meal is much more than just fuel for the body. The preparation of food is an ancient ritual that still has an important impact, not only on our health and hardness, but also our overall well-being. The stimulating effect of carefully preparing meals and then eating them should be a sensuous experience. For this to happen, the food needs to be highly appetizing with its particular aroma, color, and shape. It is understood that the meal should also abound in flavor.

I knew just the person who could help me create the meals I want you to try over the course of the next six weeks: Waldy Malouf, an award-winning master chef/co-owner of the highly popular Beacon Restaurant in Manhattan. Although it is the local farmers, growers, fishermen, and vintners throughout the nearby Hudson Valley who provide his wonderful produce, it is the magic that Waldy performs in his kitchen that gives his food substance, body, and emotion.

66 Let food be your medicine and medicine be your food.

HIPPOCRATES

In discussing my Six-Week Program with him, I gave Waldy two provisos that I wanted him to keep in mind when he created his meals:

- The entrees should be flavorful, high-energy, and easy to prepare.
- Meals should be designed with the novice chef in mind, but they must be exciting and tasty enough that people could constantly look forward to them day after day.

Waldy was intrigued by the challenge and went back to his kitchen. Several weeks later, an email arrived. Waldy had developed and tested a dozen special meals for me, two for each week of the program. Each offering provided exactly what is necessary from each of the major food groups, but was also sensuous. By sensuous, Waldy means that each contains a variety of spices that will help increase your awareness of eating as a physical pleasure—like sex. What is even better is that these meals provide the ingredients that will strengthen your Hardness Factor. With the spark and energy from these nutritious meals, I hope that you will go on to exceed all of your Hardness Factor goals.

Of course, you do not have to use Waldy's recipes **(see Appendix II)** in order to progress with the Hardness Program. If you decide to create your own recipes, take a look at Waldy's to see that eating sensibly does not mean eliminating tasty and interesting foods from your diet. Feel free also to adjust these recipes according to your own taste preferences and individual dietary concerns. Be creative and above all, enjoy each meal.

HARDNESS FACTOR SUPPLEMENTS— NATURE'S VIAGRA

Folk medicine has always been applied whenever a man's hardness showed signs of waning. A seemingly endless succession of herbal potions and mechanical devices have been employed over the centuries, from crushed rhinoceros horn and pulverized antelope, deer, and horse testicles, to parings of human nails. In times of desperation, a piece of bone was eased into the urethra to stiffen the penis.

The mandrake plant, a member of the nightshade family, was used extensively in medieval Europe, northern Africa, and Asia as both a painkiller and a hardness solution. Stemless, with bell-shaped flowers, the plant's long and thick root, which often divides into two sections, resembles the lower male torso. It contains many alkaloids of medicinal value, making it one of the most discussed plants in medical literature, as well as the subject of myth and superstition. Alkaloids are a diverse group of nitrogen—containing substances produced by plants that have powerful effects on body function; some of the more common alkaloids include atropine, morphine, quinine, and codeine.

One old American hardness recipe combined thorn apple, black pepper, and honey. This mix was applied to the penis before intercourse. The thorn apple is now known to contain atropine and hyoscine, two strong alkaloids. Absorbed through the mucous membrane of the penis, they may have helped to trigger an erection. The pepper, which produces a burning sensation, would have helped to maintain it, with the honey a lubricant.

Native Americans often used jimsonweed *(Datura stramonium)* as an erection builder. A tall, highly poisonous plant that is also a member of the nightshade family, its seeds were powdered, mixed with butter, and eaten; for added measure, the mixture was smeared on the genitals.

We have certainly come a long way from mandrake, jimsonweed, and thorn apple. During the next six weeks, I am going to recommend that you take a variety of Hardness Factor supplements—the same ones I take and recommend to my patients. Here is an overview of what I want you to use to enhance your hardness:

Pycnogenol/L-arginine. The use of antioxidants—chemical compounds that neutralize the damaging effects of cellular byproducts called free radicals—to bolster various biological functions has been recognized for years. But when I learned about the long-range benefits of the antioxidant Pycnogenol combined with L-arginine, I realized that a whole new chapter in sexual medicine was about to be written, based in part on this extraordinary pine-bark extract that enhances and protects penile hardness—as well as reduces the risk of chronic diseases.

This combination of Pycnogenol and L-arginine will directly impact your endothelium, the lining of your blood vessels, shielding them and al-

So What Did "LBJ" Stand For?

President Lyndon Baines Johnson referred to his penis as "Jumbo."

Even LBJ Was Impressed!

The late Dominican playboy, Porfirio Rubirosa, was famously endowed. His penis was said to be 11 inches long and 6 inches in circumference.

Now That's a Big Bertha

A 1999 golf tournament in Australia offered a penis enlargement to the player with the longest drive.

lowing for better nitric oxide utilization. The end result is a rock-hard erection.

Antioxidant complex. I am also going to recommend that you take several antioxidant supplements, among them vitamins C and E, resveratrol (a powerful substance that comes from red grapes), and grape seed extract, another powerful oligomeric proanthocyanidin—commonly called an OPC—that works as a free-radical scavenger in the body. OPCs are thought by some to be more powerful than vitamins E and C.

What this antioxidant complex is designed to do is protect against free radical damage and help reduce fatty deposits in the blood that can lead to diminished cellular function, impaired heart function, and reduced hardness.

Omega-3 fatty acids. I am an avowed fan of omega-3 fatty acids, which are commonly found in fish. Research supporting a cardioprotective role for omega-3s has been accumulating since the 1970s, when population studies showed that Eskimos and Japanese fishing families tended to have low rates of atherosclerosis and heart attacks.

There is now good evidence that these oils lower the risk of cardiac arrest, a life-threatening medical emergency characterized by the abrupt cessation of the heart's pumping action. The marine fish oil can reduce plaque inside artery walls, decrease blood clotting, lower triglyceride (blood fat) levels, and decrease both blood pressure and blood vessel inflammation.

Horny goat weed. A good part of my week is spent listening to patients talk about their flagging sexual desire. Many have come to see me complaining that their sex life is not what it used to be and they want to know how to initiate needed changes. Most need ways to ramp up their sexual interest.

This is where horny goat weed can certainly help. And, yes, that's really its name. Sometimes all that is needed to perk up your sex life is a little boost from this interesting Chinese herbal mixture. I recently completed a forty-five-day double-blind placebo-controlled study with Exotica, the brand of horny goat weed developed by Pinnacle, a New York–based company. This is a proprietary combination of plant parts, primarily *Epimedium sagittatum* (horny goat weed), but also including three other well-known herbal sex boosters, Lepidium meyenii, Mucuna pruriens, and Polypodium vulgare.

As an interesting historical sidenote, *Epimedium sagittatum* has been used as a sexual enhancer by the Chinese for more than 2,000 years. How horny goat weed creates sexual fire is unclear, but researchers think it may be related to its specific stimulating properties, perhaps working on the hypothalamus or pituitary gland.

Within a week of taking these herbs, my phone rings with men calling to say that whatever it is they are taking, they want to make sure the supply will not run out.

Niacin. This supplement, also called vitamin B_3, has earned a reputation as a natural cholesterol-lowering agent that often rivals prescription drugs in mild to moderate cases.

Unlike most prescription cholesterol-lowering medications, which simply lower levels of LDL cholesterol and the bad fats found in triglycerides, niacin also raises levels of HDL cholesterol. As a result, this vitamin may prove more potent than conventional medicines in ultimately reducing the risk of a heart attack.

GETTING FIT FOR SEX

The benefits of exercise for health and hardness are not a new discovery: centuries ago, Hippocrates said that when the body is unused and left idle, body parts become susceptible to disease and the body as a whole ages quickly. Hippocrates' observations—which came without benefit of the exhaustive medical research and detailed studies that we have today—are still valid.

Research has proven that working out regularly helps decrease your chance of having a heart attack or stroke by improving your circulation and metabolism. Regular exercise also lowers both your heart rate and blood pressure and helps clear life-threatening plaque from arteries by changing your cholesterol profile. This all translates to harder erections.

Of course, exercise alone—even if you run more than 50 miles a week—does not automatically grant you immunity from such life-threatening events. But research has shown that men who exercise regularly have a much lower risk of dying suddenly of a heart attack than do sedentary men.

In a celebrated study by Dr. Ralph Paffenbarger, Jr., of Stanford University, it was reported that of 17,000 male Harvard graduates (classes 1916 through 1950), those who exercised through midlife, burning at least 2,000 calories a week (the equivalent of about five hours of walking), were more likely to survive a heart attack than were their more sedentary classmates. These active Harvard men, Dr. Paffenbarger discovered, had a 31 percent lower risk of dying from heart disease than did the moderately active Harvard alumni, and a 46 percent lower risk than the very inactive.

SEXUAL FITNESS

The type of exercise we will be using in the Hardness Factor Six-Week Program is what is known as Functional Fitness. This is a series of exercises that focus on building a body capable of performing real-life activities in real-life positions. It's a type of fitness training that can reinforce one's ability to be good at a particular sport, but more important it strengthens and supports the function of the body in one's everyday life.

Functional Fitness is not about performing a series of reps while lifting a certain amount of weight in a static posture: imagine standing upright performing biceps curls with a barbell. In contrast, Functional Fitness tries to replicate the integrated play of your muscles as they really work in life—from bending to reaching, and swinging to pushing and pulling. It's the movements one makes when squatting to get a book on the bottom shelf or lifting a suitcase out of the well of a deep car trunk. Imagine performing those same biceps curls while sitting on an oversized stability ball or while standing on a BOSU board. All of your muscles will be called upon to keep you balanced as you attempt to lift the weights.

So if Functional Fitness is about learning the movements and exercises that mimic everyday situations so one can be in better shape for life, then Sexual Fitness is a series of movements and exercises that will better prepare you for one of life's best workouts—good sex. What's so good about having well-defined biceps or impressive six-pack abdominals if you are unable to maneuver or lift your lover without throwing out your back? Not much at all, unless you happen to derive a certain amount of secret pleasure from looking at yourself in the mirror.

What, then, is the best way to get in shape for sex? As you will find out over the next six weeks, the best way comes, in part, from functional exercises. These are exercises that help strengthen your body so you can perform daily activities—sex being one—without any discomfort.

The sexual fitness regimen we will be using in the Hardness Factor Six-Week Program consists of a series of exercises recommended by Jana Angelakis, a popular New York fitness trainer and two-time Olympian. From the many functional exercises available, she has carefully chosen those that closely mimic movement patterns one would expect to use during sex.

Many of these stretching and strengthening exercises are performed while lying down, and they stimulate the body's core muscles—the abdomen and lower back. The exercises, which borrow from physical therapy and yoga, also involve a soupçon of balance to challenge the nervous system. The end result is more control and total body strength and endurance. When it finally comes time to play in the bedroom—or wherever—you will be able to bend, lift, push, and pull without worry of any residual soreness or worry.

"An important characteristic of these sexual fitness exercises is that they require no special equipment," notes Angelakis. "Using nothing more than one's body weight, all the muscle groups can become better integrated, working together as a team instead of isolated strands. The best part is that anyone can start training right away, no matter what shape he is currently in."

In the Hardness Factor Six-Week Program you will slowly develop muscles that will help lower your cholesterol, shed fat, build muscle, and improve your balance, but you will also build muscles that promote stamina and help lengthen your sexual sessions. Most important of all, this total integration will aid in increasing the hardness of your erection.

PUT ON YOUR WALKING SHOES

Good sex is a physical activity and I want you to have the stamina, strength, and flexibility you need so you can truly explore your sensuous—and adventurous—side. I want you to be able to have the ability and mobility to try any sexual position without risking cramps or fatigue as you bear your partner's weight.

I am going to ask you to exercise daily over the next six weeks. As part of this program, I want you to do something every day that should be very simple: walk. Again, it was Hippocrates who once said, "Walking is man's best medicine"—and he was certainly right about that.

I have chosen walking because it uses almost all of the 650 muscles and 206 bones in the body, and also because it is a great way to shed pounds and develop muscle. Granted, most people walk no more than 6,000 steps daily. By the sixth week, I want you to have increased that distance to at least 10,000 steps a day. I will show you how to add the extra distance effortlessly. All you will need to purchase is an inexpensive pedometer to do your step counting for you.

I also want you to perform a series of sexual fitness exercises that are designed to restore and realign you, and to make you as strong and balanced as nature intended. This simple ten-minute-a-day regimen will make an enormous difference in how you feel and look. All I ask is that you put the cell phone on "silent" and give yourself the uninterrupted quality time each day. Remember, the harder the workout, the harder the erection will be.

START IT UP

I am confident that the suggestions I offer in the Hardness Factor Six-Week Program will help men live fuller, more vital lives. I've seen it happen again and again as I have worked with so many different people. But while everything that I advise is eminently doable, I don't mean to imply that it's going to be a snap.

Lifestyle changes take a considerable amount of effort. What I have done is broken the various lifestyle shifts into small steps that build upon one another as you go along, week after week. This way you won't feel overwhelmed by the process of transformation. I also discuss the thought processes behind each recommendation.

The good news I have to report is that with the Hardness Factor, you are never too young to be concerned about hardness. And you are never too old to do something about it.

It's time to make the commitment to your six-week adventure. When you do—and I hope you are ready to go as soon as possible—you will quickly find that you never felt better or harder.

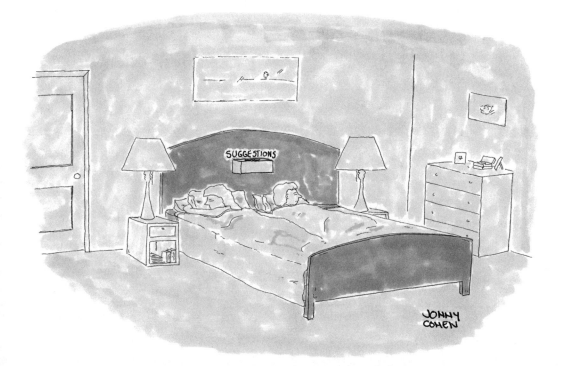

> **"** *We used to be triple-X-rated*
> *Look at us now, so domesticated*
> *What happened to babe and stud?*
> *Too much KFC and Bud*
> *I shout it out into the wind*
> *Are we ever gonna have sex again?*

"Are We Ever Gonna
Have Sex Again?"
Amy Rigby

Part Two

THE HARDNESS FACTOR SIX-WEEK PROGRAM

Hard Is Good—Harder Is Better

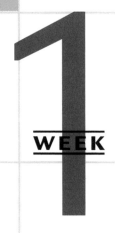

1

WEEK

For those of you not familiar with Functional Fitness, I recommend that you take some time now and go to the exercise section in this chapter. Look at the specific exercises I recommend. They are easy, manageable, and will help create a foundation on which the rest of the program will build. When you are able to perform the exercises with correct form, you will train your muscles to support your body throughout the day and night.

Also, before you begin the program, review the appropriate boxes in the next few pages to see what you will need to purchase in terms of supplements, specific foods, and a step counter (pedometer) for your daily walking.

4

BUILDING A FOUNDATION

Congratulations! Getting started with the program is often the most difficult part of the whole six weeks for many men. The best way to begin is to have your exercise and walking time already penciled in as best you can, as if you had made an important appointment for yourself. By developing this positive, simple habit you are preparing the way for profound improvement for a lifetime.

THE START OF A LIFETIME OF HARDNESS

If every great journey is accomplished one step at a time, the Hardness Factor Six-Week Program provides the all-important stepping stones that guide men toward a healthier, happier, and more passionate life. This program can certainly help men achieve these goals. Let's get started.

The First-Week Assignments

Sexual Fitness

▸ The goal is to walk every day this week. I want you to take at least 5,000 steps daily, which should not be too strenuous. If you already swim or bike on a daily basis, I still want you to get in this minimal amount of walking.

▶ I find that a step counter is an invaluable piece of equipment to own. Purchase one at your local sporting goods store or buy one on the web at *digiwalker.com* or *accusplit.com*. Compact, accurate models cost approximately $20–$30.

▶ In addition, I want you to perform each of the special sexual fitness exercises that are recommended to help get the body strong and flexible. These are the Side Lunge Reach, push-ups (Classic or Modified), and the Plank.

Hardness Factor Supplements

▶ Take 80 mg of Pycnogenol and 3 g of L-arginine once daily (Prelox Blue, Pycnogenol Plus).

Sensual Nutrition

▶ Chef Waldy Malouf offers two exciting meals I want you to try.

▶ How heavy you are will affect your sex life in just about every imaginable way, from the ability to achieve and maintain an erection, to your ability to maneuver your partner into different positions, to your overall self-esteem.

▶ This week I want to show you how to focus on foods that can enhance erections and remove foods from the diet that diminish hardness.

Hardness Factor Lifestyle

▶ Buy a body fat scale. How much weight you lose is not the best indicator of your success on the Six-Week Program because your bathroom scale can't distinguish between pounds that come from body fat and those that come from muscle or lean body mass.

▶ When you lower your body fat to safe levels through regular physical activity, you can help prevent or control the development of many life-threatening diseases. Carrying too much fat—30 percent or more of your total—is called obesity,

WEEK ONE   *WEEK TWO*   *WEEK THREE*

and it puts a person at risk for serious medical conditions including heart disease, diabetes, and even certain types of cancer. **(See Appendix III, page 317.)**

How Do You Measure Up? Body Fat Ranges for Men

- **Optimal:**   6–17 percent
- **Average:**   18–24 percent
- **Overweight:** 25–29 percent
- **Obese:**   30 percent

Special Task

- Check the medicine cabinet. Over the past decade, the pharmaceutical industry has come up with an incredible array of medications for a vast number of illnesses. Unfortunately, many prescription drugs can be the biggest erection downers, and when taken in combination may offer a KO punch to your hardness. What I want you to do is review all the medications you are currently taking and compare them to the list of drugs that impact hardness at www.thehardnessfactor.com. If any of yours are on the list, speak to your physician about hardness-friendly alternatives.

VITAMINS FOR THE PENIS—AND BLOOD VESSELS

It is certainly wonderful that we now have three prescription erection drugs in the hardness arsenal. But these are the big guns that only have to be taken out for the most serious erection problems—those caused by the nerve damage of diabetes, devastating atherosclerotic build-up, high blood pressure, and long-term smoking. Don't misunderstand me. These drugs are great and certainly get the job done. However, they do not do anything for the underlying medical condition that is causing the hardness problem in the first place.

When I was invited to take part in a combined European-American research effort of a natural supplement that would enhance endothelial health and thereby contribute to long-term heart and penile health, I gladly accepted.

The six-month study had enrolled fifty men under the age of 50 who took two blue pills a day containing the mixture of Pycnogenol (pronounced pick-nah-geh-nall) and L-arginine. The goal of the study was to determine if this combination nutritional supplement would enhance hardness and improve overall sexual satisfaction. As I was to discover, the experimental product did just that, and today it is marketed worldwide as Prelox Blue.

What the Prelox study revealed—mirroring the results of an earlier Pycnogenol/L-arginine study conducted in Europe—was that 85 percent of the test subjects who took the product on a regular basis had significantly enhanced their sex lives. DIR readings for almost every man increased significantly.

BARKING UP THE RIGHT TREE

Pycnogenol, a patented amalgam of more than three dozen antioxidants extracted from the bark of the French pine tree, has a lot of scientific research behind it. This extraordinary product can prevent or reduce the risk of chronic disease triggered by free radicals. In addition, Pycnogenol enhances blood flow to the penis, as well as to the heart.

Pycnogenol's role in improving heart health is a real attention grabber with my patients, but its ability to improve sexual function holds even more interest for men. With more blood flowing to the corpora cavernosa within the penis, the harder the penis will become. That means those who take Pycnogenol will benefit from a supplement that not only protects

WEEK ONE   WEEK TWO   WEEK THREE

vital organs, including the heart, by serving as a powerful antioxidant, but will also add to the overall Hardness Factor by maintaining maximum blood flow to the penis.

What I have come to like so much about Pycnogenol is its broad spectrum of health benefits. In addition to its powerful antioxidant effects—which help in protecting against cancer, heart disease, and other diseases linked to the chemical action of free radicals—Pycnogenol helps restore elasticity and smoothness to the skin by reinforcing collagen fibers, and it strengthens tiny capillaries, the blood vessels that help nourish cells, such as the ones in the penis.

THE PRICE WE PAY FOR FREE RADICALS

Since the groundbreaking research more than forty years ago by Dr. Denham Harman at the University of Nebraska College of Medicine, scientists have come to agree that free radicals are now linked to dozens of deadly diseases. Obliterating cells in their path and mutating DNA, they wreak havoc and weaken our body's defenses, making us susceptible to a number of killers, including cancer and heart disease.

Free to roam, free radicals have the limitless potential to negatively affect every part of our bodies—particularly the delicate tissue in the penis. In addition to the conditions it already affects, free radical damage is now being linked to hypertension, stroke, Alzheimer's disease, leukemia, Parkinson's disease, congestive heart failure, and irritable bowel disease.

PYCNOGENOL BATTLES FREE RADICALS

Thankfully, there are steps we can take to fight back. Without these strong countermeasures, free radicals would quickly overrun our bodies, abruptly ending our lives. But while our bodies do have their own built-in defense systems, the ability to combat such a continuous assault is limited.

WEEK FOUR   WEEK FIVE   WEEK SIX

My weapons of choice are antioxidants, which react with free radicals, neutralizing their detrimental effects. They work by stabilizing the molecule by donating an electron so that the free radical will leave healthy cells alone.

Extensive medical research indicates that increasing intake of certain nutrients, especially vitamins C and E, grape seed extract, and resveratrol **(see Week Four),** will help to protect against the ravages of free radicals. Pycnogenol can be a very helpful addition.

A broad-spectrum nutrient with numerous applications, Pycnogenol is unlike any other antioxidant. I choose it repeatedly as the solution to counteract free radicals and enhance the active lives of the men in my Hardness Factor Six-Week Program.

Pycnogenol Benefits

- Helps the body neutralize free radicals, which oxidize LDL cholesterol and increase its destructive effects on arteries.
- Keeps blood platelets from becoming sticky as they pass through narrowed arteries, thereby preventing them from clotting at plaque sites.
- Protects the endothelium (the cells of the heart lining), thereby reducing the formation of blood clots, which can lead to a heart attack.
- Decreases blood pressure by inhibiting the formation of angiotensin, a substance in the blood that constricts vessels.

A HARDNESS BOOSTER—HOW L-ARGININE WORKS

L-arginine is an amino acid that is one of the essential raw materials used by the body to build protein. Like the other twenty-one natural amino acids, L-arginine performs specific and vital tasks in the body. It builds muscle, assists in the release of growth hormone from the pituitary gland, fights off infections, and battles cancer. I have also found that L-arginine often improves the quality and duration of erections, making a man feel and perform like a younger version of himself.

Think of your arteries as living pipes that carry oxygen and nutrients to your body's cells. Ringing these pipes are smooth muscle cells that expand or contract to regulate the flow of blood, making sure that the proper raw materials in the right amounts get to where they are needed. This process of vasodilation (opening) and vasoconstriction (closing) in the arteries is regulated by chemical signals sent to the smooth muscle cells from neighboring endothelial cells. The signal is sent in the form of a release of nitric oxide, and the endothelium makes the NO by breaking down L-arginine.

> **O**f Course, They Also Had Tiny Feet
>
> Two British scientists conducted a study and found no correlation between a man's shoe size and the length of his penis.

During the course of your lifetime, your heart will beat roughly 3 billion times, propelling as much as twelve ounces of blood through your circulatory system with each beat. Throw in the added stresses of drinking, smoking, a diet high in cholesterol, and the increasingly sedentary nature of modern life, and you will have accumulated a significant amount of taxation upon your delicate circulatory system. As a result, your arteries lose some of their elasticity over time and it becomes increasingly difficult for them to maintain the rigorous routine of dilating and constricting in order to keep your blood flow at optimal levels.

By boosting the levels of L-arginine that are available to your endothelial cells, you provide the material they need to slow the hardening process in your blood vessels and even to reverse some of the damage already done. When L-arginine supplements are taken in tandem with a daily routine of physical activity, a synergistic effect is produced that markedly increases your production of NO. This means greater blood flow to all areas of the body and, specifically, to your penis.

By taking 3 grams of L-arginine in supplement form per day, roughly doubling the amount that men typically get from their diet, you should quickly begin to see an improvement in the hardness of your erections.

WEEK FOUR   WEEK FIVE   WEEK SIX

> 66 The arteries of the penis will actually become rejuvenated, capable of pumping all the blood needed for longer-lasting erections.

And, unlike prescription erection drugs, this is no one-night stand, no quick fix. As the L-arginine level builds in your system over time, providing those over-worked endothelial cells with ample amounts of the raw material they need to produce NO, the arteries of the penis will actually become rejuvenated, capable of powerfully pumping all the blood needed for potent, longer-lasting erections.

THE HARDNESS FACTOR
PYCNOGENOL/L-ARGININE PROGRAM

This week, I want you to begin taking 80 mg of Pycnogenol and 1 gram of L-arginine a day. On day 3, I want you to increase your dosage of L-arginine to 2 g, going to the full 3-g dosage on day 7. It is best to take the tablets on an empty stomach since protein will inhibit the absorption into the bloodstream. Most of my patients report no side effects from the supplements, but if you happen to experience minor stomach upset, ingest the tablets with a small amount of carbohydrate. For those taking Prelox Blue, take two capsules daily.

Check the Hardness Factor Shopping List **(page 325)** for recommended Pycnogenol, L-arginine, and Prelox Blue choices.

Pycnogenol/L-arginine Benefits

- Helps men achieve and maintain an erection more easily.
- Improves sexual responsiveness and drive.
- Naturally supports blood flow to the sexual organs.
- Quickly absorbed into the bloodstream.
- Supports circulation and cardiovascular health.
- Can be used daily by men of all ages.

WEEK ONE   WEEK TWO   WEEK THREE

Pycnogenol: New Hope for Harder Erections

PETER, age 35—A study in hardness

A messenger arrived at my office with a handwritten note from the wife of Peter, a 35-year-old subject in my ongoing Pycnogenol/L-arginine study. The advertising executive already had exceptional DIR scores in the low 2,000s. I was initially curious as to why his wife had sent me a note.

I opened the envelope and read, "Peter has become a changed man after being in your study for the past few weeks. Whatever it is in the product, it's working too well. I can't keep up with him. I want some of these pills for myself!"

In addition to enhanced sexually stimulated erections, Peter's nighttime erections had also increased. As I later explained to Peter in my office, these erections occur during rapid eye movement (REM) sleep, when most dreaming occurs. Generally, we experience four intervals of REM sleep per night. These spontaneous erections are the body's automatic way of keeping the "plumbing" in good working order (3 to 5 erections nightly, each lasting up to 30 minutes) and are caused by specific neuroreflexes that are stimulated during REM sleep to bring more oxygen-rich blood to the penis.

Thanks to this supplement, in addition to these increased nighttime erections, Peter also noted more sexual dreams and fantasies, and he found it easier to initiate sexual activity.

WORK OUT OR STRIKE OUT

The simple equation I want men to remember is this: Regular physical activity equals better sex. There is a definite connection between being physically active and sustaining a hard erection. The converse is just as true: If

HARDNESS FACTOR 6 WEEKS
Tone Deaf

A 35-year-old musician was unaware of any hardness problems, but his baseline DIR readings of 765 and 802 (**DIR Avg. 783**—I expected at least 1,200) had me concerned that he was on a downward spiral. Six weeks on the Hardness Factor Program saw a near doubling of his hardness to 1,389 and 1,402 (**DIR Avg. 1,395**). He felt that the addition of physical activity and supplements to his lifestyle played a major role in increasing his hardness.

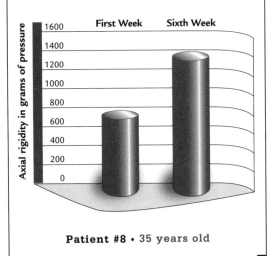

Patient #8 • 35 years old

you are not physically active, you will be throwing cold water on your sexual performance and will never achieve maximum hardness.

What regular physical activity does so well is improve cardiovascular function, which then raises the blood supply to the penis during intercourse. This will help bring about and sustain a firm erection. In addition, physical activity also positively affects brain wave activity, which makes you feel energized and vital.

Regularly working out also builds stamina, preventing or delaying fatigue during sex. Start performing my suggested sexual fitness exercises this week and you will augment muscle strength, helping to heighten sexual response, a definite asset since orgasm requires considerable muscle activity.

Finally, regular physical activity boosts testosterone levels, leading to a heightened interest in sex. As for body image, once you begin to pare away body fat over the next six weeks, your personal attitudes about sex are doubtless going to change for the positive. Even if you already belong to a gym (and actually use it), or if you are a daily runner, cyclist, or swimmer and have a set workout routine, I don't want you to substitute your workouts for the specific sexual fitness exercises I want you to perform over the next six weeks.

There are several activities I want you to include in your daily regimen this week: walking, stretching, and resistance exercises using your own body weight. These are measures that I have found to best enhance and maintain suppleness of movement as well as flexibility and strength. All activities are easy, do not require special equipment, and do not cost anything, except for the small amount I have recommended you spend for a lightweight step counter to measure your daily walks.

WALK YOUR WAY TO HARDNESS

Your goal for the Six-Week Program is to walk at least 10,000 steps a day, which, depending on stride length, is anywhere from four to five miles. I hope I do not scare you off with that distance, but stick with the program and I guarantee that by Week Six you will have no trouble accomplishing this goal. For those of you who already exercise, *regularly,* push yourself harder—and do the walking as well. You will be surprised by the gains in fitness.

Why 10,000 steps? Research has determined this is the number of steps that will get you moving enough to bolster overall fitness and health, and knock off excess weight as well. And when the weight goes down, erections go up and stay up.

One study reported that people who took fewer than 5,000 steps per day were more likely to be obese, while those who covered at least 9,000 steps were often at a very good weight. A recent study in *The New England Journal of Medicine* noted that those people who walked a minimum of 2.5 hours a week cut their risk of heart attack and stroke by one-third. I am going to ask you to walk much more than two hours a week, so you should expect your health benefits to be even greater.

Walking not only enhances endurance by increasing lung capability, it improves the strength and efficiency of muscles in the abdomen, back, and legs. In just a few weeks, daily walking can also decrease

> 66 A recent study in *The New England Journal of Medicine* noted that those people who walked a minimum of 2.5 hours a week cut their risk of heart attack and stroke by one-third.

blood pressure by as much as 10 points—it does so by improving the body's sympathetic nervous system—and by lowering blood pressure, overall penile hardness is enhanced.

Walking is the perfect long-term physical activity. It is the best activity for getting into good cardiovascular condition and maintaining it for the rest of your life. Pleasurable, alone or with a partner, it is also easy on your joints—no aches and pains when you are done for the day.

WHY WALK ?

You are probably wondering why I would pick such a nonstrenuous activity as walking for the preferred physical activity in the Six-Week Program. There are several important reasons:

> **D**on't Get Scared **Stiff**
>
> Ithyphallophobia: The fear of having, seeing, or thinking about an erection.

- It is quantifiable. How many steps you take each day will help determine your overall health, fitness, and hardness.
- You will lose weight. You can burn approximately 400 calories for every 10,000 steps. By the end of six weeks it can easily turn into a loss of four pounds or more, depending on your current weight and walking speed.
- It is easy to add more steps to your day, increasing health benefits with every stride.
- Walking requires no special equipment, save for a comfortable pair of shoes and a step counter.

THE HARDNESS FACTOR WALKING PROGRAM

Walking is a good road to health and hardness. Your goal this week is to take 5,000 steps a day. If you were to make this a nonstop effort, it would take you about 35 to 40 minutes, depending on your current fitness level and stride length.

WEEK ONE   WEEK TWO   WEEK THREE

If you find it difficult to reach 5,000 steps because it is just too fatiguing, take your current walking distance and add an additional 2,000 steps as your daily goal for the next day. This is approximately a mile more of walking, but something you should be able to accomplish with two 10-minute walking sessions. By the end of the week, I expect that you will be at the 5,000-step daily pace.

If you are not in good physical condition, I want you to start with an easy stroll—about one to two miles an hour—and gradually increase your steps and time throughout the week. You do not have to walk nonstop for 30 minutes to get the full health advantage. Movement counts. Even short 5- and 10-minute intervals throughout the day will yield nice health dividends.

WALKING PACE

For those of you who do not want to use a step counter, here is a way to get a good approximation of your walking speed and distance. First, go for a walk and count how many steps you take per minute. Compare those results with the table below. These calculations are based on a 2.5-foot stride length.*

STEPS PER MINUTE	MINUTES PER MILE	MILES PER HOUR
70	30	2
90	24	2.5
105	20	3
120	17	3.5
140	15	4
160	13	4.5
175	12	5
190	11	5.5

* If your stride is longer, closer to 3 feet, then count how many steps you take in a minute and divide this number by 30. If you are taking 105 steps per minute, you are walking at a brisk 3.5-mile-per-hour clip.

EVERY STEP COUNTS

A step counter is a simple miniature device, a little bigger than a quarter, that is clipped onto the waistband of your pants when you awaken and taken off at night. Start walking and it digitally registers each step that you take throughout the course of the day. Think of a step counter as a personal "movement motivator." Counting your daily steps is a constant reminder to get more movement into your busy day. Instead of driving a car or taking a bus, the step counter will remind you to walk instead.

Once you come to realize how inactive you really are, you will quickly start to find ways to get more steps into your life.

Getting Fit Is Hard(ening)

■ ANDREW, age 34—A strained libido

"I knew that having that plaster cast on my leg would slow me down," complained Andrew, a 34-year-old insurance company executive. "But I didn't think its effects would last after I took it off."

He was referring to the aftereffects of reconstructive surgery on a snapped Achilles tendon, the result of sprinting to first base in a summer softball game. I pointed out that once he started his resistance training using his own body weight and increasing the length of his daily walks to build up stamina, the powerful muscle outline on his legs would return. He was going to make a full recovery. But something else was bothering Andrew.

"Actually, I've slowed down a lot in the bedroom, too," he admitted. "Before the accident, things were great between Sue and me. We had sex several times a week, and we both looked forward to it. It's been a very important aspect of our marriage—and we've been together going on ten years. But in the last few weeks, it has all seemed to change. Okay—since the surgery I've put on ten pounds. That I can take care of; but I'm a lot more concerned that somewhere along the way my sex drive seems to have vanished."

When he listened to my diagnosis of his lost libido—no exercise in almost two months was sure to reduce a sex drive—his face brightened considerably.

"Regular exercise equals better sex," I reminded him. Since Andrew was prevented from performing his regular exercise routine of running and weight training, it seemed to have put a crimp in his interest in sex.

Taking 10,000 steps would certainly help, as would the daily resistance and stretching exercises. And while these exertions would not help him in his preparations for his NYC marathon run in five months, they would certainly aid in revving up his sex drive.

WEEK ONE   WEEK TWO   WEEK THREE

Andrew took my advice. Three weeks later, a much-relieved man sat in my office. "You were right," he reported. "I may not be back to competitive speed when I run, but I'm where I want to be with Sue. The best thing about your 'prescription' is that I'm using my body to heal myself."

HEART-BREAKING LESSONS

Lesson 1   Sex drive is affected by medical and psychological factors.

Lesson 2   Sexual interest and ability to achieve hard erections can be independent of each other, but they can be affected equally by physiological issues.

STRETCHING YOUR LIMITS

To promote flexibility—the ability to use muscles and joints through their full range of motion—I want you to perform one specific stretch every day this week. Regular stretching also helps to relieve stress, a major contributing factor to hardness problems. When performed in a slow and focused way, stretching can be an excellent relaxation therapy as well as a tension easer.

The Side Lunge Reach will help keep the muscles used during sex limber and flexible, which will help facilitate a pleasurable sexual experience. This stretch can be performed on a firm mattress or on a mat placed on the floor. Wear either loose clothing or nothing at all. See the Side Lunge Reach on page 88.

The correct way to avoid injury when stretching

▶ Stretching should be gradual and relaxed.

▶ Do not stretch until it hurts. If there is any pain, stop.

▶ Do not bounce when you stretch; this will damage the muscle tissue.

▶ Do not hold your breath as you stretch.

▶ Breathe in through your nose and out through your mouth.

SEXUAL FITNESS

Muscle fatigue during sex is often an unwanted presence. Push-ups and the Plank are beneficial exercises to add to the weekly routine because they strengthen the shoulders, chest, and abdominals, all of which are utilized during sexual activity. Keeping these muscles strong—by using only your body weight for resistance—helps increase strength and stamina, adding to prolonged, more pleasurable sex. In the end, these basic exercises will help change the way that you feel and move for the rest of your life. **(See pages 80, 88.)**

Quick Self-Test

So, you think you are ready for some physical sex? To measure the current state of your muscles, get down on the floor.

>>You need good arm and shoulder strength for many sexual positions. See how many push-ups you can do in a minute. A man in his 20s should be able to perform at least 25. A 30-year-old should be able to manage 20.

>>Much of a man's strength and stability comes from his core, his midsection—not just the abdominal muscles, but also the lower back muscles, whose major role is to help us stand and sit without falling over. To test your midsection strength, see how many Abdominal Crunches you can perform in a minute. Lying on the floor with knees bent, feet flat on the floor, and arms crisscrossed over your chest, curl up until your shoulders come off the floor. Then return to the starting position. I expect a man in his 20s to be able to do anywhere from 40 to 50 crunches in a minute. A 30-year-old should be able to accomplish at least 40 in 60 seconds.

WEEK ONE   WEEK TWO   WEEK THREE

SENSUAL NUTRITION

What you eat and how much you eat certainly play a key role in weight maintenance and weight gain, but in the Six-Week Program I am not going to have men eating specific foods or counting calories. Rather, what I focus on instead is a combination of healthful, sensuous eating and regular physical activity as a way to trigger weight loss while enhancing health, enjoyment, and hardness.

Over the years, I have found that eating plans depending on fat grams, protein and carb counting, and deprivation just do not work. Sure, men can lose weight and improve their health profile, but after a while, the weight all comes back, and then some, and the health profile typically changes for the worse, yet again. What I want you to do instead is eat an interesting, healthful diet. Cut back on how much you eat and get in your daily physical activity, and you are guaranteed to lose the extra pounds in the upcoming weeks without even realizing it.

In the last two decades, the correlation between nutrition and optimum performance has become better understood. Guess what? Your sexual performance is greatly impacted by what you consume and how much you consume. Fatty, high-calorie foods may taste great, but they are not kind to erections. The fats injure your blood vessels to the point where they are stunned, preventing them from being reactive when sexual

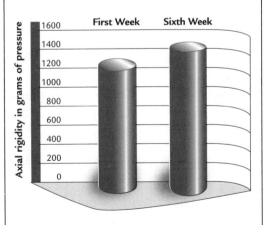

HARDNESS FACTOR 6 WEEKS
Roller Coaster

The 39-year-old overweight and out-of-shape electrician admitted being anxious about his sexual performance. Although capable of high DIR readings **(1,312 grams at baseline),** the "hard-soft" roller-coaster effect he noticed during lovemaking had him concerned. Six weeks on the program yielded a 13-pound weight loss, a substantial increase in self-confidence, a nice boost in hardness (DIR readings of 1,420 and 1,503; **DIR Avg. 1,461**), and an end to his "roller-coaster" erections. "Hard the whole time," he said.

Axial rigidity in grams of pressure

First Week   Sixth Week

1600
1400
1200
1000
800
600
400
200
0

Patient #63 • 39 years old

signals are being sent from the brain, down the spinal cord, and through the pelvis to the penis.

When it comes to what you eat, I emphasize five nutritional steps for optimal hardness and I want you to adhere to them as best you can. Beginning to incorporate these basic guidelines this week will start you on the path to enhanced hardness.

1. Reduce the Fats in Your Diet

There are many reasons why a high-fat diet is to be avoided. The main reason is that fatty foods lead to heart disease and poor cardiovascular function. Clogged arteries prevent adequate blood flow from reaching the penis, which then diminishes optimum hardness. A reduced-fat diet, on the other hand, can dramatically decrease cholesterol levels, and even reverse some of the damage already done to your arteries.

2. Sensitize Your Blood Vessels and Nerve Endings

Elevated cholesterol in the blood blocks circulation in the small blood vessels of the body, including those in the penis. Penile nerves lose their sensitivity when cholesterol builds up. Since dietary cholesterol comes mainly from animal sources, cut back on saturated fat culprits such as egg yolks, butter, cream, fatty red meats, and a variety of oils, especially those made from palm and coconut.

3. Combat Vascular Disease with Fruits and Vegetables

Fruits and vegetables have been shown to help lower cholesterol levels, which helps combat cardiovascular disease and improve blood flow to the penis. They also supply many key nutrients your body needs for optimal performance. Leafy green vegetables are excellent sources of folic acid, calcium, magnesium, and zinc. Fresh citrus fruits offer plenty of vitamin C. Asparagus, long considered a sexual stimulant in cultures around the world due to its vague resemblance to the penis, is, in fact, a rich source of vitamin E, calcium, niacin, and other minerals.

4. Eat Whole Grains, Nuts, and Seeds

A diet high in fiber and starch provides an important basis for cardiovascular and penile health. Consumption of whole grains, nuts, and seeds will add both fiber and complex carbohydrates to the diet. This can reduce the risk of heart disease and contribute to improved hardness; in addition, whole grains tend to be more filling, which can aid in weight management.

5. Spice Up Your Foods

Certain spices can contribute directly and indirectly to sexual pleasure and performance. Chili peppers stimulate the nervous system, making us sweat and causing our faces to flush and our heart rates to rise, which simulates the effects of sexual arousal. Ginger has long been considered a sexual stimulant and overall tonic for general health. Because it stimulates the metabolic system, ginger warms the body, which explains why it has long been used as a sexual aid.

HARDNESS MEALS

This week, I want you to cut back on consuming huge portions of food. I also want you to pay close attention to what you eat. The good news is that improved hardness is nothing more than a supermarket trip away. I also want you to spend more time in the kitchen preparing your meals.

Acclaimed chef Waldy Malouf believes that when it comes to cooking and eating, there are two distinct types of men: one is comfortable in the kitchen, will follow a recipe until he understands it and then change ingredients if need be to suit his taste. The other man enjoys eating but does not want to have anything to do with purchasing, preparing, or cooking his food.

Waldy notes, "Men should have fun in the kitchen. Plus, it is very romantic to prepare and cook a dinner with your partner and then share the meal together."

The expression "you are what you eat" takes on a completely new meaning when men follow the suggested meal plans I have worked out with

Waldy. The key to these sensuous meal suggestions is that they keep the saturated fats down, which is heart- and penis-healthy. As he has done with all the recipes for the Six-Week Program, Waldy has also added a variety of spices to expose the palate to new and exciting taste sensations.

66 The man who doesn't cook is missing out on one of life's true pleasures.

"My goal in creating these hardness recipes was to use foods rich in antioxidants, such as tomatoes, pineapple, peaches, figs, and salmon," he says. "I am looking for high-flavor profiles, foods that have a 'sexy' mouth feel so there is some intrigue to them, a historical aphrodisiac quality to them, whether that really exists or not. These are low-fat recipes but they still offer a great sense of adventure that is sure to spark a man's imagination."

---

*Here are two of Waldy's special entrees
I would like you to try this week*

MENU ONE

HERB-CRUSTED SALMON WITH HORSERADISH BREAD SAUCE

Chilled Yellow Tomato Soup
Herb-Crusted Salmon with Horseradish Bread Sauce
Chocolate Angel Food Cake with Brandied Strawberries

MENU TWO

**SEA SCALLOPS ON ROSEMARY SKEWERS
WITH TOMATO-GINGER CHUTNEY**

Roasted Asparagus with Scallions
Sea Scallops on Rosemary Skewers with Tomato-Ginger Chutney
Figs with Madeira and Orange Zest
(See **Appendix II** for recipes)

PLEASURE POINTS: TRAIN HARD, PLAY HARD

Men need to understand all of the components that constitute their "maleness." A major part of this program is not only making your penis harder, but making your body more aware and more alive. As your body becomes harder over the next six weeks, as your circulation improves and you become stronger and more flexible, you will also be enhancing the sensitivity of your penis. When you try these different recipes, you will also be expanding your palate, as you open yourself to the sensual world.

> 66 Foods that have a "sexy" mouth feel so there is some intrigue to them, a historical aphrodisiac quality to them, whether that really exists or not.

As you get in better physical shape, when you quit smoking or drinking excessively, when you really start to take care of yourself, life will become richer. Life itself will become the biggest pleasure point of all.

VISUALIZATION—A POWERFUL PREVIEW

Great sex occurs when you prepare. This includes what and where you are going to eat, and where you are going to have your sexual encounter. Leave nothing to chance. Most of all, you have to put your body and mind into the "zone."

How do you prepare for an upcoming sexual encounter, especially if you failed miserably in a previous effort and don't have the greatest confidence level? The natural inclination is to question yourself. My message to you is this: Don't question anything. You have to let go of the past and focus on the present and the future. Set yourself up for success. Turn off your cell phone. Give yourself enough time to succeed.

Sex is a physical act and just as athletes will practice visualization techniques so they can perform optimally, so too can you incorporate the same techniques to ensure that your bedroom performance enhances your confidence every time.

Researchers have explored human performance capabilities, and evidence increasingly points to the fact that in addition to physical preparation, mental preparation is a critical ingredient for success. Only by reinforcing mental skill can your performance be raised to the highest level.

Also called imagery or imaging, visualization is one of the easiest mental training techniques to learn. Imagine a lovemaking session, seeing with the "mind's eye." Go over every detail, from dressing, undressing, and kissing, to caressing, intercourse, and afterward. This mental rehearsal makes use of all the senses. In essence, it is simply a re-creation of experience in the form of pictures, images, and feelings that you create. Instead of telling yourself repeatedly that you will perform well in bed, you take time to imagine yourself doing this, creating a clear mental image of yourself having sex.

The human brain is incapable of distinguishing between something that actually happened from the same action that was imagined. When you vividly imagine yourself getting ready for sex, staying calm and relaxed, your central nervous system becomes programmed. It's as if the activity you've visualized has already happened. In addition, when the actual lovemaking session begins, mentally prepared men are not surprised by anything that does occur because they've seen it countless times—in their minds.

A VISUALIZATION EXERCISE

It is important to be relaxed when performing the following visualization exercise. Use this two-step technique to help learn how to relax and then visualize.

Relax: Put on music that instills a sense of tranquility. Lie on your back on a mat with your arms at your sides and take a deep breath. Hold it for a moment and then exhale. Lie still and continue breathing slowly.

Visualize: Once you are fully relaxed, picture yourself about to have sex. Patiently go through the step-by-step sequence of events. You should imagine every aspect of the session, including the sights, sounds, and smells associated with sex. Try to rehearse the action just as you would actually perform it, with the same rhythm and tempo. It's all careful practice of the ideal way you would like things to be. In the hours before a sexual encounter, mentally rehearse strategies and specific skills you will use. And when the time comes for the actual moment, your confidence will be high.

*B*ig Fingers?
Big Pointer?

Greek researchers in Athens now report that the length of a man's index finger accurately predicts the length of his penis. The scientists measured penis length in 52 healthy young males between the ages of 19 and 38 and compared it with other body measurements including height, weight, body mass index, index finger length, and waist/hip ratio. Their interesting finding, reported in the medical journal *Urology:* The length of the index finger correlated significantly with the length of the flaccid, stretched penis.

SIX-WEEK PROGRAM

1. HARDNESS FACTOR

Rate your current level of hardness for Day Seven of the program. (Check off one box.)

○ Soft   ○ Soft/Hard   ○ Hard
○ Very Hard   ○ Like a Steel Beam

2. SEXUAL FITNESS

Perform these three exercises for Sexual Fitness in the morning and again at night.

1. The Side Lunge Reach

A great total-body stretch and strengthening exercise for the adductor (inner thigh), abductor (hip area and outer thigh), core, lower back, quadriceps, buttocks, and hamstrings.

▶ Stand erect with feet slightly apart, toes pointed forward.
▶ Contract your abdominal muscles.
▶ Keeping your right leg straight, take a large step sideways with your left foot, toes pointing forward.
▶ Bend your left knee.
▶ As you lunge to the side, bend your torso over and toward your left thigh.
▶ Reach down and touch your left foot with both hands.
▶ Return to the start position by pushing off your left foot to straighten your leg.
▶ Repeat the exercise with your opposite leg.
▶ **Perform 10 times with each leg, alternating legs with each repetition.**

2. The Classic Push-Up

This exercise strengthens the muscles of the chest.

▶ Lie facedown on the floor with your legs together.
▶ Place your hands shoulder-width apart, palms flat on the floor, fingers pointing forward.
▶ Take a deep breath in, then exhale and press your whole body off the floor as a unit (from your hands to your toes) while keeping your abdominal muscles tight and drawn in.
▶ Inhale and bend your elbows as you slowly lower your chest to within 3 to 6 inches of the floor.
▶ Pause for 1 second.
▶ Push back up to the starting position and repeat.
▶ **Perform 3 sets of 3 push-ups.**
   NOTE: If you have difficulty performing three Classic Push-Ups, perform the Modified Push-Up version instead.

Modified Push-Up

▶ Lie facedown on the floor, bend your knees, and cross your ankles.
▶ Place your hands shoulder-width apart, palms flat on the floor, fingers pointing forward.
▶ Take a deep breath in, then exhale and press your chest off the floor while keeping your abdominal muscles tight and drawn in.
▶ Inhale and bend your elbows as you

slowly lower your chest to within 3 to 6 inches of the floor.

▶ Pause 1 second.

▶ Keeping your back flat, abdominals drawn in, and, using your knees as the pivot point, push your torso away from the floor as you straighten your arms.

▶ **Perform 3 sets of 5 push-ups.**

3. The Plank

This seemingly easy exercise is not that easy, and it improves core abdominal strength and endurance.

▶ Lie facedown on the floor.

▶ Place your palms and forearms flat on the floor, shoulder-width apart and parallel to each other.

▶ With your legs straight, press your entire body as a unit off the floor, balancing between your forearms and your toes. Hold this position for 30 seconds.

▶ Slowly return to the floor.

▶ **Rest for 15 seconds and repeat 3 times.**

3. WALKING

Take 5,000 steps a day. Circle each day you achieved this goal:

Sunday   Monday   Tuesday   Wednesday
Thursday   Friday   Saturday

4. HARDNESS FACTOR SUPPLEMENTS

Pycnogenol/L-arginine
Take Pycnogenol (80 mg)/L-arginine (3 g) mix

5. SENSUAL NUTRITION

Fish

As a practicing physician, I recommend having fish at least one to two times a week. Here are some easy, flavorful recipes that will make you look forward to fulfilling your fish prescription.

Prepare two sensuous meals this week:

▶ Herb-Crusted Salmon with Horseradish Bread Sauce

▶ Sea Scallops on Rosemary Skewers with Tomato-Ginger Chutney

A MAN @ 15

Effortless, uncontrollable, extremely hard erections with minimum or no apparent stimulation.

Ejaculations occur with minimum stimulation.

A capacity for repeated erections and ejaculations.

Needs to understand all issues that will affect his long-term health and hardness.

An important period for developing sexual awareness; early sexual experiences can have a critical impact on future sexual life.

145–135 degrees

THE PENIS & THE PROTRACTOR

There are no two identical men and therefore, no two identical penises. The numerous anatomical differences that may affect the angle of erection make it difficult to produce a clear-cut classification of "good" or "bad" angles of erection for different age groups. However, this chart aims to indicate the angles created by the erect penis (from the legs upward) throughout various age groups. Please note that individual penile size, girth, and shape will all have an influence on the angle of an erection.

Head 180 degrees

Feet 0 degrees

DEGREES OF AGE

THE FIRST WEEK—NOT SO HARD

You are on the way to making significant changes in your life, reversing patterns of behavior that were not good for your health or hardness. Now that the first week is over, write down a schedule noting the how, when, and where for next week. You'll get far better results when you are able to sketch out your plan of action for the week.

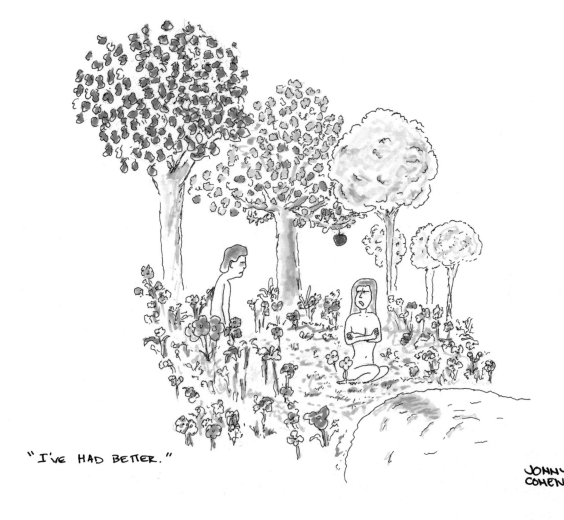

"I've HAD BETTER."

JOHNNY
COHEN

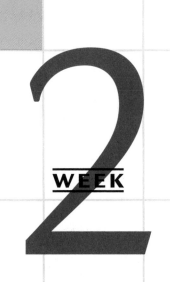

WEEK 2

Continue your exercises for Sexual Fitness from last week and get ready to add some new ones to the routine. Your walking distance will increase by another 1,000 steps. As you will see, it's not a big jump, but if you have been inactive, you may have to find ways to get in the extra distance. For instance, if you play golf, walk the nine or eighteen holes. And always take the stairs whenever you can. Walking up and down stairs is a great mini-workout for your legs and heart.

5

THE HARDNESS FACTOR LIFESTYLE

Be honest: It wasn't very difficult last week. If you weren't able to complete the full number of repetitions for some of the exercises, try to complete them all this week. Cut back on idle snacking this week, and you will see the pounds start to drop. Commit yourself to more improvement over the course of the next seven days.

ENDURING HARD TIMES

A constant presence throughout our lives, libido ebbs and flows as much as the tides. Springing from an intricate network of physiological and psychological components, libido varies from man to man. Certain hormones play a role in sexual feelings and sexual activity. The most influential is testosterone, sometimes called the libido hormone.

The Second-Week Assignments

- The first week was probably novel and interesting for you and you were determined to succeed. In the second week, like many types of courses, the program may lose some of its novelty and may even seem a little tougher as you take it up a notch.

▶ Be careful this week. It may be easy to come up with excuses to not follow through with some of my suggestions. But they are just that: excuses. For those of you who like taking notes, you may want to jot down your thoughts in a training diary. *Progress is made when progress is measured,* so each night review your day's achievements. This will not only motivate you to adhere to the program, but by the end of the remaining five weeks, you may be very surprised to see how far you've come along.

▶ If you weren't able to complete the full number of repetitions in some of the exercises last week, aim to finish them all this week. Keep up your walking; you may notice that it seems slightly easier. To avoid boredom on your daily jaunts, consider walking in the opposite direction.

Sexual Fitness

▶ Increase your daily walking by 1,000 steps. Increase your push-ups to 3 sets of 5 Classic or 8 Modified. In addition to the Side Lunge Reach, begin performing the Angry Cat Stretch and the Cobra.

Sensual Nutrition

▶ Drink some black or green tea as a morning beverage or as an accompaniment to your meals.

Hardness Factor Supplements

▶ Start taking 2 horny goat weed supplements daily with your dinner. Each capsule should contain at least 500 mg of horny goat weed.

Who Has Time for a Libido?

TOM, age 32—The ups and downs of a career

Tom was unhappy, yet again. Divorced for the past four years and eager to remarry, this dapper 32-year-old office-supply salesman had been looking for one woman he could be happy with both romantically and sexually. "Yet again, a great woman, great potential, but the chemistry changed," he said to me, describing a ten-month relationship that had just hit a bad patch. "It was probably my fault that Charlotte had to continually initiate sex. It's not that I wasn't interested; I just didn't have her sex drive and couldn't keep up with her. I began to feel awkward and embarrassed. How do you explain it?"

Tom cared deeply for Charlotte, but in the past two months, he admitted that his interest in sex had slowly ebbed away. He had recently been promoted at work and began traveling more, returning home exhausted. Sex was not on his mind like before and he started to come up with excuses to sidestep Charlotte's familiar advances. Not understanding why this was happening, but feeling the pain of rejection, Charlotte finally told Tom she felt they needed a break, that perhaps they should not see each other for a while. "I want to feel like a woman should feel," she told him.

Tom is far from alone in questioning just what triggers a man's sexual appetite. Springing as it does from an intricate network of physiological and psychological factors, sexual chemistry—that elusive spark that ignites a man's desire and puts him in the mood for sex—varies from man to man. And woman to woman.

In Tom's case, Charlotte, who was five years younger, had a much higher libido as well as expectations of more frequent sexual encounters. Not getting nearly what she needed sexually made her unhappy and caused problems in their relationship.

I told Tom that his case was not very unusual. In our fast-paced world, a healthy sex life is often lost as men desperately try to keep up with other demands as they move up their career ladder.

Although no one is certain why one person has a stronger sex drive than another, neuroscientists are just beginning to unravel and better understand the chemistry of sex. They are coming up with answers to what exactly makes us tick—and what can help us tick even better.

In Tom's case, libido was simply sidetracked by his career ambitions. While his blood levels of testosterone were well within the normal range, his sexual focus was blunted by his all-consuming desire to do well in his job. I recommended that if he really wanted to save his relationship with Charlotte that he refocus his life and find the time and energy to be intimate with her. Charlotte probably wanted nothing less than to feel wanted, desired, pampered, appreciated, worshipped, and loved. It was up to Tom to show her that he really cared.

Since he was in a sex-starved relationship that was totally of his own doing, I recommended that he schedule fewer office-related functions and put more effort into Charlotte—even if it meant scheduling a date. Another suggestion was a sex night with each other, with the phone switched off, household matters ignored, emails unchecked, and absolutely no talk of office matters. Total focus was to be on each other during this "planned spontaneity."

I also handed Tom a bottle of Exotica horny goat weed capsules and told him to take two daily, plus another four an hour before an anticipated sexual encounter. Tom gave me a quizzical look but said he would take them as directed.

Tom cared for Charlotte and was more than willing to do whatever it took to restore their relationship and get Charlotte back into his life for good. He left the office with the bottle of horny goat weed tucked in his pocket.

With his sex life ebbing, Tom started to take steps to keep it from spiraling downward even more. Making sex a higher priority in his life was an important positive step. He took his horny goat weed supplement, which he later told me triggered the most vivid sexual dreams he ever had. He and Charlotte also began setting up "sex dates"—an evening set aside when they spent time together as a couple. Three months later, Tom was back to see me, along with Charlotte. They looked like a couple in it for the long term.

"The sex dates certainly helped set the mood," Tom admitted, "and brought about the healing between us. Little by little, I got my spark back. It's great being with Charlotte. Our nights are wonderful, both physically and emotionally."

Charlotte was beaming. She showed me her engagement ring. "He's a new man, Doctor. I can't thank you enough."

CAREER LESSONS

▶ **Lesson 1**   Most men are distressed by a decreasing interest in sex.

▶ **Lesson 2**   Sexual drive can be an important barometer of a man's physical and psychiatric state.

▶ **Lesson 3**   Depression, stress, and anxiety are significant inhibitors of libido.

HALFHEARTED SEX RESULTS IN HALF-HARDNESS

Men expect to be thinking about sex, if not all the time, then at least a good part of the day. It is part of who we are. Moreover, if we are not thinking about sex, then our minds are wandering, as a patient of mine once told me.

When desire for sex starts to diminish or sex suddenly begins to lose its familiar piquancy, many men are quick to point an accusatory finger at their partner. However, more often than not, most causes of a lagging libido have to do with a man's lifestyle and health and not very much with his relationship. When nothing can get a man fired up for a lovemaking session—a romantic setting, a sex-laden whisper, a fragrance—then a closer look needs to be taken to find out why.

This week I want you to focus on bolstering your interest in sex. Later on, I will tell you more about the very interesting herbal compound that has the power to make you as randy as a goat. However, before I get to that, I want to discuss libido, the appetite for sex. If your libido seems to be waning, the cause is often temporary and directly related to your lifestyle.

Enacting my suggested changes this week will certainly help raise libido a notch or two, maybe even three. For starters, are you walking, taking your 6,000 steps daily? Physical activity stokes the fires of lust. Have you cut back on the fats and transfatty acids in your diet? Eating more of the right foods takes the emphasis off your stomach and puts it in your loins. By examining your lifestyle and making the few changes that I recommend, you will find that your appetite for sex will be restored.

> **H**ere Comes the Judge!
>
> In 2004, an Oklahoma City judge was accused of using a penis pump and masturbating while sitting on the bench.

LET'S GET LUST

When two people do hit it off, it has a lot to do with chemistry. Among the key factors in sexual functioning and libido are the neurotransmitters dopamine and serotonin. These two important brain chemicals send messages to the nerve cells and play a positive role in determining our sex drive.

Dopamine, nestled deep in the brain stem, is the "pleasure" chemical messenger that makes us feel good, the all-important ingredient in sexual arousal. Researchers believe that it's our dopamine system that is ultimately responsible for evaluating and rewarding the various sensory stimuli we encounter in the course of the day. As sensory information—what we smell, hear, taste, touch, and imagine—comes into the brain from the outside world, sensory states are produced.

For example, when a man sees someone attractive, the brain, which has collected numerous memories and experiences of such encounters, immediately transmits this information to the dopamine system, which then sets the stage for possible action. If there is a possible reward—say, a weekend away together—dopamine is released, triggering a sexual spark.

However, if the moment is not "right" ("I'm too stressed out from work to think about anything but going to sleep") or if there is little expectation of reward ("I didn't brush my teeth") then the red light goes on and no dopamine is released. Normally, dopamine pulses on and off as needed, but in some, the "go ahead" release of dopamine is less frequent than in others, resulting in low libido.

Serotonin is dopamine's foil. It is clearly a calming neurotransmitter that has a significant effect on our moods, aggression levels, and sensitivity to pain, as well as which foods we seek and how much of them we eat. Serotonin levels are now positively linked with several common disorders. Too little serotonin, for example, can lead to imbalances affecting mood, sleep, and food consumption.

On the other hand, too much serotonin can have decidedly negative effects on your sexuality, so maintaining the correct balance is critical. For example, when an antidepressant medication such as Celexa, Effexor, Lexapro, or Serzone is taken, serotonin is released and the brain levels are subsequently raised. This can have several positive effects, including relief from depression. The drugs, however, may also cause hardness problems. Many of the treatments for psychiatric-related disorders negatively affect sexual response by affecting the autonomic nervous system, which controls the genitals. Other drugs can block nerve function, making it difficult, or even impossible, to achieve an erection or ejaculation. High doses of tranquilizers, prescribed for anxiety and depression, not only cause

> **F**ill 'Er Up
>
> The amount of semen produced with each ejaculation is 1–2 teaspoons. The typical man will produce about 14 gallons of semen throughout his lifetime.

hardness problems, they can also be responsible for the lessening of sexual desire or an inability to ejaculate.

While it sometimes happens that hardness and sexual problems diminish after a man has adjusted to the drug he is taking, it is usually the exception to the rule. Taking a "drug holiday" on the weekend or having sex when the drug is at its lowest concentration in the body are alternatives that work for some men.

Be sure to speak to your doctor if you are experiencing hardness problems after you begin taking a particular antidepressant. Do not stop the medication on your own and do not reduce the dosage of the medication on your own.

We also know that libido is clearly linked to testosterone, the primary male sex hormone. This all-important hormone creates sexual desire, lust, and hunger for sex. Let's examine this hormone a little closer and see how it works in the body throughout a man's life.

You've Lost That Lovin' Feeling

A.J., age 51—Rub and make a wish

Barbara was upset, almost to the point of tears. I handed her a tissue and she continued her story about her 51-year-old husband of one year. "A.J. has just about lost all interest in me and our sex life. He says nothing is wrong, but Doctor, I know there is a problem. I don't think he finds me attractive anymore. I don't know how else I can explain it."

Drops in libido can be linked to "male menopause" or "andropause," as it is often called. Nomenclature aside, it all has to do with changes in mood, weight, bone density, muscle mass, energy level, and libido triggered by a drop in natural testosterone levels.

Testosterone, an androgen (male sex hormone), is a hormone derived from cholesterol. It is produced primarily by the testes, but the signal to produce it comes from the pituitary gland, in the form of two other hormones, which arrive in pulses at certain times of the day. As men age, the response of the testes becomes more muted; for men older than 40, the levels of testosterone in the bloodstream decline, on average, by a little more than 1 percent each year. It is now believed that as many as one-third of the men in the United States have low levels by the age of 60.

"The loss of desire in a man can be troubling and very difficult for a woman to accept," I said. "When a man who has always been ready and able to perform in bed is now suddenly not interested, it's not uncommon for the partner to think it's perhaps due to diminished physical attraction or bedroom skills. But it could be that A.J.'s levels of testosterone may be dropping quicker than normal for a man his age," I said. "But I would have to check to be sure."

I told Barbara about the study I was conducting with thirty test subjects who were using AndroGel, a rub-on colorless testosterone gel that men with low testosterone levels rub on their shoulders each day. Not only did many of the men boost their testosterone levels in less than thirty days, from below the limit of normal up into the normal range, but their levels of sexual desire and penile hardness, as measured by the DIR, jumped with it. Barbara brightened a bit after I told her this.

"Will you please talk to A.J. about this study?" she asked. "And is there any room in the study for him?"

"I'd be happy to speak to him," I said. "One of the most common reasons for loss of sexual desire, and with it, penile hardness, is a low testosterone level. Barbara, your job is to get A.J. to come and see me. Do that, and if, after running some blood tests, he meets the criteria for testosterone replacement, I will invite him to join the AndroGel study. That's a promise."

"A.J. has his pride, you know. What exactly should I say to him so he will come to see you?"

"Here's all you have to say," I told her. "It's a thirty-day testosterone study of men that may reveal changes in fat loss and gains in

The Goldilocks Complex

According to the Kinsey Institute's studies on sexuality, when women are troubled by penis size, it's because the penis is too big rather than too small.

muscle strength. Men can relate to that. It should be enough to get him interested."

A.J. was in the office three days later to sign up for the AndroGel study. I drew blood to measure his testosterone levels (A.J. was later found to be below normal). Testosterone levels decline slowly with age but the impact is not as dramatic as the sudden loss of estrogen in women.

Between age 60 and 80, for example, more than 20 percent of men have levels less than the low level of normal testosterone, with upward of 5 million men in this category.

A.J.'s blood test showed a testosterone level of 285 nanograms per deciliter of blood (ng/dl). Typical normal ranges for testosterone are between 399 and 1,000 ng/dl.

Although he surely wasn't completely testosterone deficient, A.J. was definitely on the low side. He had no evidence of abnormalities that could be contributing to his low levels—such as testicular or prostate cancer, pituitary disease, or cirrhosis of the liver—so I recommended that A.J. join my ongoing testosterone replacement study.

After he signed the study consent forms, I explained how this powerful hormone could enhance muscle growth and fat loss, and possibly boost his libido, the desire to have sex. A.J. said nothing when I mentioned this, which I found surprising. "How is your sex life?" I asked.

"Fine."

"Is your wife happy with it?" I asked.

"Yes."

I also explained to A.J. that the increase in testosterone in his system might cause him to think of sex more often and might even increase his number of sexual encounters over the next few weeks. He might even find that his penile hardness increased, too.

"Fine. If it happens, I will be sure to report it," he said, as he walked out the door with the study forms in his hand.

TO BE CONTINUED ▶

ESSENCE OF A MAN: TESTOSTERONE

Testosterone is an androgen, one of the masculinizing hormones that lead to muscle tissue development, lowering of the voice, and overall growth. It also affects libido, memory, and lean body mass, and it may contribute to mood issues and irritability.

Contrary to popular belief, testosterone is not exclusively a male hormone. Women make a tiny bit in their ovaries and adrenal glands, and it plays an important role in sparking their sexual passion. Men produce testosterone in their testes; they have far higher levels of testosterone in their systems than women do, about fourteen times more.

At birth, baby boys have testosterone levels that reach those of young adult males. They drop quickly, however, and remain low until puberty, when they begin to rise, masculinizing them in the process. Hormone production continues to rise, tapering off at about the age of 40.

Some men have insufficient blood levels of testosterone, a condition known as testosterone deficiency. As a man ages, the amount of testosterone in his body naturally drops off to lower, but still normal, levels. Some scientists label this decline "andropause" or "male menopause." Other causes of testosterone deficiency that may drop testosterone to lower and suboptimal levels include the following:

> **G**ive 'Em an Inch
>
> A boy's penis typically starts growing at age 11 and stops at age 17. The average length of a flaccid penis is 3.5 inches. When erect, the average length ranges from 5.2–6.4 inches.

▶ chemotherapy

▶ injury to the testicles

▶ pituitary gland abnormality

▶ medication (certain antidepressants)

▶ alcoholism

▶ any chronic illness

▶ stress

WEEK FOUR   WEEK FIVE   WEEK SIX

Testosterone levels are almost never static. Throughout the day, testosterone rises and falls. Some researchers think there is an hourly difference as well, which might explain men's preoccupation with sexual thoughts.

NEED A LIFT?

Over the past few years, I have boosted the sagging testosterone levels of many of my male patients with testosterone replacement therapy. The effects have been uniformly remarkable and the men have gone on to have satisfying sex lives. The long-term effects of testosterone supplementation on healthy males are still not known, and may not be for years to come. For some men, increased testosterone may cause prostate growth, a risk for men with an already enlarged prostate or undetected prostate cancer. Any man using testosterone replacement therapy needs careful monitoring by his doctor.

IT'S NOT JUST A GUY THING

I have found that women have always been more proactive about their health than men. Many are also more proactive when it comes to their sexuality. This was recently brought to the fore when the expected approval by the Food and Drug Administration (FDA) of a female sex drug was surprisingly overturned.

There is currently serious debate about the safety of a testosterone-based drug for women suffering from a form of "female sexual dysfunction" linked to low levels of sexual desire. Although it's thought of as an exclusively male hormone, testosterone is not exclusive to men. Testosterone, as it does for men, plays a vital role in sexual desire levels in women. Generally speaking, women have about 5 to 10 percent as much testosterone as men.

However, when the much-anticipated quality-of-life testosterone patch for women was in its mandatory testing phase, concerned doctors questioned the relative importance of sexual relations and an orgasm juxtaposed against the possibility of long-term—and heretofore unknown— health problems caused by chronic testosterone treatment. These problems could entail not only acne, a deepening voice, and facial hair, but possibly heart disease and stroke.

Many women were upset that the FDA, the national watchdog of drug safety, had delayed the approval of this novel testosterone treatment, recommending instead even more testing by the drug company behind the drug. I heard from many women suffering from the loss of libido who were annoyed with the FDA decision. "I was ready to take that risk of possible future health problems," said one patient. "I want my sex life back. A healthy sex life is what I don't have and now it appears I won't have it for quite some time."

The complete role of testosterone in women still isn't known. What is understood is that, for some post-menopausal women, a decline in testosterone can cause thinning pubic hair, declining libido, and a reduction in overall muscle mass.

While you are using testosterone, your physician should check your progress during scheduled visits, especially during the first few months of treatment. The dosage may have to be finely adjusted. My male patients are monitored regularly, and I check their prostate glands for signs of enlargement, a possible side effect of testosterone supplementation. I also examine women systematically for any signs of virilization, marked by a deepened voice, acne, or facial hair. However, at such low levels, I have not witnessed any of these changes. Follow-up blood levels of testosterone may also be helpful in guiding therapy.

TESTOSTERONE CHECKLIST

Testosterone production declines naturally with age. However, testosterone deficiency can occur because of damage to the hypothalamus, pituitary gland, or testicles, which plunges testosterone levels to suboptimal levels. Insufficient testosterone production can lead to loss of libido and abnormalities in muscle and bone development.

Check off any symptoms of low testosterone you may be experiencing:

1. Do you have a decreased sex drive (libido)?
   ○ **Yes**   ○ **No**

2. Are your erections less hard?
   ○ **Yes**   ○ **No**

3. Do you have a lack of energy?
   ○ **Yes**   ○ **No**

4. Do you have a decrease in strength and/or endurance?
   ○ **Yes**   ○ **No**

5. Have you noticed you are losing height?
   ○ **Yes**   ○ **No**

6. Have you noticed a decreased enjoyment of life?
   ○ **Yes**   ○ **No**

7. Are you sad and/or grumpy?
   ○ **Yes**   ○ **No**

8. Have you noticed a deterioration in your ability to play sports?
   ○ **Yes**   ○ **No**

9. Are you falling asleep soon after dinner?
   ○ **Yes**   ○ **No**

10. Has there been a deterioration in your work performance?
   ○ **Yes**   ○ **No**

NOTE: If you have one or more of these symptoms of low testosterone, contact your doctor immediately.

WEEK ONE   *WEEK TWO*   *WEEK THREE*

STRESS: THE LIBIDO KILLER

Another factor to consider when evaluating the lust level is stress. When stress levels start to rise, as they did for my patient Tom, testosterone levels and the desire for sex typically start to decline.

Financial worries, long hours at the office, moving along on the career path, and concerns about raising children and taking care of elderly parents all push sex far from center stage in many men's lives. People under stress may experience such symptoms as headaches, backaches, rapid heartbeat, fatigue, difficulty sleeping, recurrent nightmares, irritability, or a loss of concentration.

Many people tell me that they are too stressed and tired to make love, and as sexual frequency starts to drop, this becomes a major source of conflict between partners. In most of these sex-deprived relationships, all the genital equipment is often in fine working order. The root cause is generally psychological and linked directly to stress, the often inescapable daily annoyances of life.

For the most part, stress can diminish the number of sexual encounters by dampening sexual arousal. Arousal, which includes a surging of blood, increased heart rate, and penile erection, depends in great part on a number of various hormones (most important—testosterone) to play their specific roles.

There are also hormones that can effectively shut down the sexual response as well. For instance, there is adrenaline, a hormone that adversely affects libido. Whenever a person is under stress, no matter the source, adrenaline starts to course through the veins, directing blood flow to the

---

A Hard Luck Case

A man walks into a bar and sees his friend slumped over the rail. He walks up and asks what's wrong.

"Well," the guy says. "You know that beautiful girl at work that I wanted to ask out, but I got an erection every time I saw her?"

"Of course," his friend replies with a laugh.

"Well," says the guy, straightening up, "I finally got the courage to ask her out, and she agreed."

"That's great!" says the friend. "When are you going out?"

"I went to meet her this evening," the guy continues, "but I was worried I'd get an erection again. So I got some duct tape and taped my penis to my leg, so if I did, it wouldn't show."

"Makes sense," says his friend.

"So I get to her door, and I ring her doorbell. She answered it in the sheerest, tiniest dress you ever saw."

"And what happened then?"

The guy slumps back over the bar again. "I kicked her in the face."

---

heart and major muscles—away from the genitals—preparing them for a "fight or flight" response. Both heart rate and blood pressure increase in the process. This reaction is a genetic inheritance from our ancient ancestors, who experienced a similar sensation whenever they came face to face with a charging beast.

> 66 Stress can diminish the number of sexual encounters by dampening sexual arousal.

The modern response to psychological stress is no different, only it can lead to emotional outbursts if there is no way to defuse it. Too much unrelieved stress can cause hypertension and other heart diseases. Even a small amount of outside pressure can shut off our sexual impulses. Studies with soldiers preparing to head into battle have proved it. Testosterone levels plummeted when the soldiers were facing their enemy, only to rise again after their return.

WARNING **Contents Under Pressure**

Although the inclination to have a couple of drinks or a bowl of vanilla ice cream when under stress is understandable, it is a mistake to rely on alcohol or comfort food as a means of coping with stress.

▶ Destructive behaviors such as overindulgence in alcohol or smoking can magnify the effects of stress and may contribute to sustained increases in blood pressure. Here are three suggestions that can reduce stress and boost energy.

▶ Make sure you get your 10,000 steps a day. Walking helps clear the mind. Even 1,000 steps, a ten-minute walk, can decrease anxiety levels. As you walk, beta-endorphins are released. These are the body's natural relaxants that counteract the stress surging through your body. Besides offering a well-needed break in your daily routine, walking gets blood circulating, boosts your mood, and eases tension.

▶ Call a friend. A sympathetic ear can help lighten the load. Researchers have found that having good friends helps lower blood pressure, relieves anxiety, and may even help you live longer. Many experts list friendship as the key factor in getting through stressful times. Do not isolate yourself, as many men often do. One fifteen-minute session with a good friend might be all that's needed to make you feel better.

▶ Don't bring work home on the weekend. Leave work on Friday without a briefcase. Even if you need to go in early on Monday, having a weekend free of job pressures is enough to help relieve built-up stress.

MEN AND MASTURBATION

"What can I do?" said Fred, a handsome 29-year-old executive. "My wife was stunned. I was in the shower when she happened to pull the curtain back and saw me masturbating. It's something I have been doing a few times a week, ever since our twins were born. Of course, I was doing it a lot less before the children came along, but that's because Jacqui and I had been having sex several times a week. Now, she's just too tired for anything. Who can blame her? She's got her hands full from morning to night. But I have my needs, too."

Fred is certainly not an anomaly, nor is masturbation—sexually stimulating oneself—abnormal or harmful as it's been described throughout the centuries. In fact, it's quite normal. I explained that men (and women) masturbate, whether they are young or old, unmarried or married. Some masturbate more often than others, some rarely or not at all. While most men engage in "solo sex," many are ashamed or embarrassed to talk about it since it's an activity that historically has been surrounded by ignorance and shame and cited as the cause for most of the world's evils.

Dr. John Harvey Kellogg, a talented and dedicated staff physician at the Battle Creek Sanitarium in Michigan, did his best to help prevent men from harming themselves through masturbation by advocating circumcision and creating a new breakfast cereal, corn flakes, in the early 1900s. Strange as this was, even stranger was the fact that Dr. Kellogg also opposed sexual intercourse, never made love to his wife, and lived in a separate residence from his wife throughout their marriage.

Masturbation is common, whether a man has a regular sex partner or not. According to *The Janus Report on Sexual Behavior,* a detailed survey of the sexual activities of Americans published more than a decade ago, several interesting facts were reported:

- 44 percent of married men masturbate at least once a week
- 48 percent of single men masturbate on a weekly basis
- 68 percent of divorced men masturbate daily or weekly

Even with the historic taboo and guilt surrounding self-stimulation, masturbation is slowly losing its stigma and is oftentimes viewed by men as a panacea for a host of medical complaints, ranging from stress and anxiety to sleeplessness and depression.

Since men are the best experts on the function of their own bodies, pleasuring themselves also allows them to know that, in lieu of sexual intercourse, they can still get hard; it's a quick and easy way to regularly gauge their hardness and ejaculatory potential. One of my patients, Ron, the 31-year-old artist, readily admitted to me that on several occasions he had masturbated as much as ten times daily, just as a hardness self-check. "That's what my father did, too," he told me proudly.

Some of my patients with premature ejaculation will often masturbate a few hours before a possible sexual encounter with their partner as a way to "desensitize" their penis, allowing for longer sexual activity before reaching orgasm when they have intercourse.

I explained to Fred that he was a vital, sexual being and that he needed to talk to his wife. Since Jacqui now knew her husband's "secret," I encouraged him to explain that masturbation was not a substitute for sex with her. Rather, it was his way of meeting personal physical needs that were currently not being satisfied in the relationship, since she was too fatigued from childcare to engage in their regular sexual activities.

I also recommended that during this time they might consider developing a new sexual scenario for themselves in which masturbation played an important role. Pleasuring himself in front of her or having her do it for him would keep them from becoming estranged sexually and possibly emotionally, and could help solidify their bonds of intimacy and caring.

HIGH BLOOD PRESSURE = LOW LIBIDO

Men with hypertension are typically concerned that their hypertension medication will dampen their sexual desire and negatively influence overall sexual performance. However, a recent study suggests that the problem may not lie with the blood pressure medications so much as with the primary impact of high blood pressure on the body—and erections.

Researchers studied men in their 40s who had recently been diagnosed with hypertension. These men were healthy and were not taking any type of medication. They were then compared to a similar group of men who did not have high blood pressure.

The scientists found that those men with hypertension had much lower levels of sexual activity than men without elevated

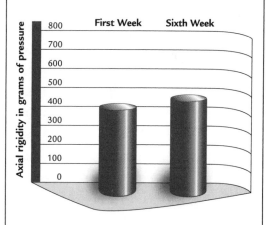

HARDNESS FACTOR 6 WEEKS
Sexual Medicine Is a Good Thing

The 45-year-old dentist had severe hypertension and diabetes and should have been on the program at least a decade sooner. DIR readings of 395, 409, and 406 **(DIR Avg. 403)** were consistent with his underlying chronic ailments. Six weeks of the program yielded a 15-pound weight loss and the elimination of one hypertension medication but only a minimal boost in hardness (468, 488, and 491 DIR readings—**DIR Avg. 482**). While he said he would continue with the program, he would also add a prescription erection drug to the regimen before sex to ensure maximum hardness.

First Week   Sixth Week

Axial rigidity in grams of pressure

800
700
600
500
400
300
200
100
0

Patient #G-38 • 45 years old

blood pressure. In addition, they had significantly lower testosterone levels.

So, which comes first, the lower libido or the hypertension? No one is sure of that answer just yet. However, it is safe to say that if you have elevated blood pressure, take your hypertension medication. In addition to protecting you from heart attack and stroke, it may just help restore your libido as well.

HORNY GOAT WEED MAKES YOU, WELL, HORNY

This week I want you to start taking two horny goat weed capsules daily. Granted, it is a strange name for a supplement, but behind the funny name stands a time-tested herb that increases libido and bolsters hardness. Known in China as Yin Yang Huo, horny goat weed *(epimedium sagittatum)* has a 2,000-year history of use as a libido enhancer. In ancient Chinese texts, the leaves of this plant were described as the primary food of a mythical animal that achieved a hundred sexual climaxes daily, and the herb still holds an important place in traditional Chinese medicine. Today, it is gaining popularity around the world as more men discover its power as a libido enhancer.

> 66 Behind the funny name stands a time-tested herb that increases libido and bolsters hardness.

How powerful is horny goat weed? Several years ago, I was surprised when I went to a study investigator's meeting for a national clinical study that was about to be launched with Viagra. My job was to enroll in the study thirty men with complaints of erectile dysfunction. Over the course of the study, I was to note what impact Viagra had on their sexual satisfaction. There was a caveat, however. No man in the six-month trial could use horny goat weed because it might skew the study results.

HORNY GOAT WEED AND SEXUAL SATISFACTION

For my first clinical study with horny goat weed, I wanted to see if it had prosexual effects on healthy men. I also wanted to see if it boosted the libido of men with mild to moderate erection problems who needed to use Viagra to achieve a suitable erection. I also enrolled a third group of healthy men in the study as a control group, and I told them that the pills they were given might boost their libido and enhance their erections. What I did not tell these men was that the pills were placebos and would have no biological effect whatsoever on their libido or erections.

I have to admit that at first I was a bit skeptical about an herb being able to increase sexual thoughts and dreams in men, but after reviewing the data at the end of the study, it was clear to me that horny goat weed was definitely doing something to my study subjects. Many of the men told me of their amazing increase in libido and sexual dreams. At the end of the study, most asked if they could keep any extra capsules they still had.

In this study, I reported that the Pinnacle brand of horny goat weed (Exotica), which contained 500 milligrams of horny goat weed, did enhance sexual satisfaction in 60 percent of healthy male subjects and 45 percent of men using Viagra. The placebo had no impact at all. My interest was piqued, and I soon conducted another study with the Chinese herb.

A year later, I wanted to see if horny goat weed had a positive effect on hardness in sexually active male volunteers looking to enhance their hardness and sexual performance. The men in the study were not told what the product was that they would be taking, only that it might or might not help increase libido and erection hardness.

For this study, I used the Digital Inflection Rigidometer. This was the first study of its kind anywhere in the world where the hardness factor was objectively measured after taking an herbal supplement.

In this study, I reported that taking four horny goat weed capsules one hour before sexual activity resulted in a significant increase in hardness in two-thirds of the healthy male subjects.

THE HARDNESS FACTOR
HORNY GOAT WEED PROGRAM

Take 2 horny goat weed capsules daily. Make sure that the product you purchase has **500 mg of horny goat weed** (*Epimedium sagittatum*). One to two hours before a possible sexual encounter, **take 4 additional capsules for an extra libido boost.** I recommend the Pinnacle brand of horny goat weed, Exotica, because I know I can depend on its quality. Each year, Pinnacle Company president Mel Rich has his agents go to the herb markets in Bozhou, China, to select the best horny goat weed. The leaves of the plant are picked wild on the slopes of Tianmu Mountain, located in a national nature reserve in western Zhejiang Province.

In addition to horny goat weed, Exotica also contains 250 mg of maca *(Lepidium meyenni),* a sex-enhancing herb from the highlands of Peru, and 33 mg of Mucuna *(Mucuna pruiens),* a popular Indian herbal remedy for men and women with low libido. I want you to take this supplement **on a daily basis for the next two weeks.** Once you come to appreciate its stimulating effects, you might find its optimal use when used on an intermittent or "as needed" basis for the rest of the program.

Check the Hardness Factor Shopping List **(page 327)** for recommended horny goat weed choices.

Skipping Dessert for the Main Meal

JAY, age 38—Horny goat weed at the beach

One of my horny goat weed study participants, Jay, relayed the following story of his experience with the randy herb. On a vacation trip to Cape Cod, Jay took four horny goat weed pills shortly before his dinner at a local restaurant. He never made it to the dessert course. "Midway through the meal," he said, "my wife looked at me with total surprise and whispered, 'You're acting like you did when we were engaged.' "

She was right about that. "The horny goat weed was very powerful," said Jay, with a broad smile on his face. "I got a 1,900 gram reading on the DIR after taking the horny goat weed. Luckily, it was off-season at the hotel and no one was in the room next to ours. We made a lot of noise that night. Like goats."

HIV

Thanks to new prescription non-nucleoside reverse transcriptase inhibitors, men with HIV (human immunodeficiency virus) are now living longer, leading fairly normal lives, hoping one day to be cured of their disease.

The sex lives of men with HIV are definitely not over as long as they practice safe sex. Many, unfortunately, do have problems with libido, orgasm, and hardness. Due to muscle wasting caused by HIV, men are often prescribed human growth hormone to preserve muscle mass and sexual function. With a drop in testosterone due to some of the medications they may be taking, many are also prescribed testosterone replacement therapy—with a drug such as AndroGel—to boost abnormally low testosterone levels. Prescription erection aids, such as Cialis, Levitra, or Viagra, are also prescribed for those men with moderate to severe erectile dysfunction.

I strongly recommend the Hardness Factor Six-Week Program to all men, including those living with HIV. Not only will the program make them healthier, it will enhance their hardness so they can put a condom on and practice safe sex.

MAKE TIME FOR TEA

Need something to wash down your horny goat weed capsules? I am a longtime fan of tea—and for good reason. Tea is one of the most potent health drinks we have. From maintaining heart function and bone strength to cancer protection, a hot cup of tea has too many disease-fighting benefits to be ignored. So, whenever my patients ask what meaningful changes they can make in their diet, a recommendation to drink tea every day is always made. This week, I want you to drink some tea.

Tea is good for you, so why not switch off from coffee on occasion, taking a tea break every now and then this second week of the program? Drink black, green, or white tea, or the type found at your local grocery store. Whether you want loose tea leaves, tea bags, or bottled, the choice is yours. I happen to enjoy the Fuze brand of bottled tea. Steep loose tea in 6 ounces of water that has been brought to a rolling boil for 2 to 5 minutes to make sure the full complement of antioxidants are released. Research from Holland reports that the addition of milk to the tea will not block the antioxidant release.

---

*Here are two new Waldy Malouf recipes
I want you to try this week*

MENU ONE

SUMMER VEGETABLE RISOTTO

Sweet Tomato and Mozzarella Salad with Grilled Scallions
Summer Vegetable Risotto
Peaches with Balsamic Vinegar and Roquefort

MENU TWO

**CHILI-RUBBED CHICKEN FINGERS
WITH MOLASSES AND BRANDY SAUCE**

Shrimp with Tomato Horseradish Salsa
Chili-Rubbed Chicken Fingers with Molasses and Brandy Sauce
Caramelized Bananas with Blood Oranges, Rum, and Spices
(See **Appendix II** for recipes)

A.J. and Barbara:
Back to That Lovin' Feeling

Barbara and A.J. sat together in my office as I reviewed A.J.'s AndroGel study diary. A.J. had lost significant body fat in the thirty days he had taken the medication. For a man who put in ten-hour days at work most of the week, he appeared vital and well rested, another possible side effect of the testosterone boost.

I could tell from a brief look at the diary that A.J.'s sexual appetite had increased during the past four weeks as well, peaking in the last week with four sexual encounters with Barbara. His hardness figures, as measured by the DIR, pointed to a significant jump from 900 grams of pressure to more than 1,500 grams, a steel beam.

"Well, what do you think, A.J.?" I asked. "Do you notice anything different over the past four weeks?"

"If you had asked me four weeks ago if I thought having sex once every month or so was okay, I certainly wouldn't have disagreed with you," A.J. said. "I didn't miss the sex at all. It's like when you lose your appetite. I never really missed something that I never missed, if you know what I mean. Not having sex became like a habit for me. However, the way I feel now, that wouldn't seem all right for me. And especially not for Barbara."

Barbara smiled. "It's been like we were dating again, Doctor," she said.

"I don't think that's fair," A.J. said, straightening himself up in his chair. "I didn't love my wife any differently before. It never changed how much I enjoyed being with you, the fun, and the excitement. I've always been crazy about you. It's just that other things were on my mind. The sexual part of me just slowly slipped away and I wasn't aware of it."

"How do you think the AndroGel affected your life?" I asked.

"After the first day of using the drug, I felt a different kind of vibe in my body that I hadn't felt in a long time. Using another food analogy: it was as if I had not been hungry for a long time and suddenly placed before me was a four-course meal consisting of my favorite foods. I started salivating. I felt hungry again.

"What the drug did was remind me of my sexual side. It also made me realize how much fun sex is and the important role that it plays in my relationship with Barbara. Looking back, I can't understand how I could ever have forgotten this."

"Testosterone is interesting," I told the couple, "in that it works on libido to allow a man to perform well sexually. When testosterone levels decrease, so does sexual appetite. This usually happens as a man ages, but not in the same way as a woman's libido decreases due to menopause.

"A man can have an active and healthy sex life well into his 70s and beyond. Testosterone is the male hormone that works to keep a man's sexual desire normal. Any change in testosterone levels will cause a change in libido, as it did over time for you, A.J."

A.J. wanted to know if he needed to use the AndroGel for the rest of his life.

"What you will have to do on a regular basis is have a blood test to monitor your testosterone levels and a PSA test to track any changes in your prostate," I told him. "You may find that you will have to continue with the drug indefinitely. Did you find that using the gel was uncomfortable or difficult?"

"Not at all," A.J. said. "It was no problem. Just one more thing to do in the morning. Along with my bifocals and arch supports, and the Lipitor for my cholesterol, it's really not surprising that I would need something like this."

A.J. and Barbara clasped their hands together. "We are so grateful, Doctor," Barbara said. "A.J.'s back and we have a whole new world to explore together."

TESTOSTERONE LESSONS

Lesson 1 Pharmacological agents, both prescription and natural, can have a dramatic impact on libido.

Lesson 2 Healthy men have a normal waxing and waning of sexual interest.

WEEK FOUR   WEEK FIVE   WEEK SIX

SIX-WEEK PROGRAM

1. HARDNESS FACTOR

Rate your current level of hardness for Day Fourteen of the Program. (Check off one box.)

- ○ Soft
- ○ Soft/Hard
- ○ Hard
- ○ Very Hard
- ○ Like a Steel Beam

2. SEXUAL FITNESS

FROM WEEK 1:
- The Side Lunge Reach (10 repetitions)

1. The Angry Cat Stretch NEW
This exercise actively stretches your lower back.
- Get on the floor on your hands and knees, with your hands shoulder-width apart, fingers pointing straight ahead.
- Tuck your chin in toward your chest, contract your abdominal muscles, and round your back up toward the ceiling. Make sure your back is curved, starting at the base of your skull to your tailbone.
- Hold the rounded back position for 10 seconds.
- Relax your muscles and return to the start position.
- **Repeat 3 times.**

FROM WEEK 1:
- Classic Push-Ups (3 sets of 5 reps) or Modified Push-Ups (3 sets of 8 reps)
- Plank (3 sets: hold 30 seconds, rest 15 seconds)

2. The Cobra NEW
Think of this as a two-for-one exercise that stretches your core and increases the flexibility of your spine.
- Lie on your stomach with your face almost touching the floor.
- Place your palms on the floor, at the sides of your shoulders.
- Keep your legs together and the tops of your feet resting on the floor.
- Push up, bringing your head off the floor.
- Keep your pelvis pushed into the floor while relaxing the buttocks as best you can.
- Slowly arch your spine backward, straightening your elbows.
- Bring your head back and look at the ceiling.
- Hold the position for 3 seconds.
- Descend slowly to the floor.
- **Repeat 10 times.**

3. WALKING

Take 6,000 steps a day. Circle each day you achieved this goal:

Sunday Monday Tuesday Wednesday Thursday Friday Saturday

4. HARDNESS FACTOR SUPPLEMENTS

Take Pycnogenol (80 mg)/L-arginine (3 g) mixture or Prelox Blue.

Horny Goat Weed (2 500-mg capsules) NEW
Take 2 horny goat weed capsules daily. Take 4 capsules one to two hours prior to a sexual encounter.

5. SENSUAL NUTRITION

Tea:
A cup of tea per day has many health benefits. How many cups of tea did you have this week?
○ None   ○ 1–3 cups
○ 4–6 cups   ○ 7 or more cups

Vegetables, Grains, and Chicken:
Research has consistently shown that people who consume a diet high in vegetables, fruits, and grains have a reduced risk of heart disease and many types of cancer. As for chicken, you couldn't ask for a better low-fat protein source—a simple, smart choice for a hardy meal.

Prepare two sensuous meals this week:
▶ Summer Vegetable Risotto
▶ Chili-Rubbed Chicken Fingers with Molasses and Brandy Sauce

A MAN @ 25

Period of peak physical strength, speed, flexibility, and endurance.

For many men, the most sexually active period of their lives.

High sex drive, capacity for multiple erections with minimal stimulation.

Multiple orgasms still possible.

Stress and relationships starting to affect hardness.

Premature ejaculation can be common and needs to be addressed.

May be noticing erection quality issues due to lifestyle (little physical activity, smoking, drinking, lack of sleep).

135–120 degrees

THE PENIS & THE PROTRACTOR

Head
180 degrees

Feet
0 degrees

DEGREES OF AGE

THE SECOND WEEK—STARTING TO GET HARD

As you start to see signs that you are making progress, you will be motivated and inspired to continue with the program. When you can see that you are becoming more flexible and physically stronger and that your libido has been boosted, your desire to make even more progress is increased. You are becoming empowered by your actions, more self-confident through your successes. Commit yourself to making yourself stronger, healthier, and harder. Embrace the process and make it part of your new way of living.

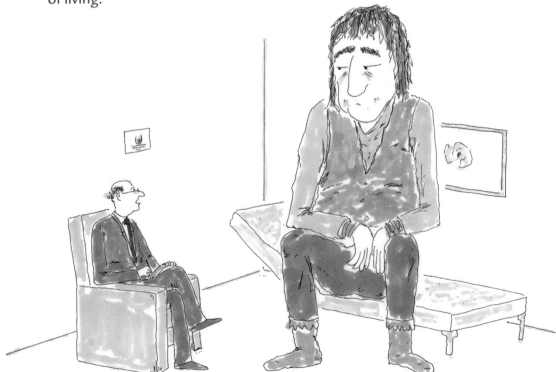

"WELL YES, THEY DO SAY SIZE DOESN'T MATTER."

JONNY COHEN

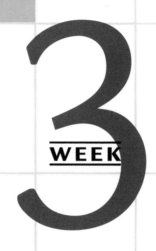

3

WEEK

Most of us are sleep deprived, which affects our health and hardness in subtle, but often dramatic ways. I know we could all use more sleep, so this week aim to get to bed no later than 10:30. You may feel odd, even guilty, for getting under the covers at that time but with the extra hours of high-quality sleep, you will soon notice the benefits—consider it an evening vacation. With the body able to fully restore itself as you sleep, you will feel rested, more alert, productive, and happy.

6

THE HALFWAY MILESTONE

Goals are the rocket fuel for your motivation to improve your health and hardness. At the end of each week's chapter in the program, you have been checking off your weekly goals, your achievements for the previous seven days. It's these goals that have kept you walking 6,000 steps a day when you felt like stopping a few thousand short. Goals have made you push and strain through push-ups and side lunges. Goal-setting has encouraged you to change what, how much, and when you eat. Writing down the new personal goals that you want to achieve increases the chance of success. If your goals are not in writing, they're only wishes. Tracking your goals is the first step toward achieving them.

RENEW YOUR HARD RESOLVE

It's a milestone and an important one, too. You're halfway through the program. If you have been following my suggestions for the past weeks, I am certain that you have come a long way. You deserve kudos and praise. But then, maybe you're thinking about quitting. Perhaps you feel that you've already done enough. You are happy with your gains and want to stop the program.

My advice is straightforward: Banish those thoughts. You have to be more responsible. You owe it to yourself and your partner to continue with the program for the next three weeks. Sure, it may not be easy. But don't stop now. As men get older, we often have the tendency to coast, to pull back and not give a complete effort. One shouldn't coast in life. Be strong. Be proactive. If you are hard now, you are going to be even harder—and healthier—three weeks from now.

The Third-Week Assignments

Sexual Fitness

▶ Increase your daily walking by another 1,000 steps, bringing the total to a minimum of 7,000 steps this week. Add Squats to your body-resistance program and the Woodchopper Stretch to stretch out your upper and lower body.

Hardness Factor Supplements

▶ Start taking 2 omega-3 supplements daily. Each capsule should contain at least 300 mg of DHA and 400 mg of EPA.

Sensual Nutrition

▶ Increase your lycopene intake this week.

HARDNESS FACTOR SUPPLEMENTS— OMEGA-3S ARE #1

Cardiovascular disease is the number one killer of men (and women, too) in the United States. For that reason, doctors have been searching for years for heart-protection breakthroughs. Now it appears they may have finally found one called EPA and DHA (eicosapentaenoic acid and docosahexaenoic acid). We know them better as omega-3 fatty acids. Omega-3s are a specific type of polyunsaturated ("good") fat, and they are found in abundance in oily fish such as salmon and sardines. Marine fish oil supplements are also an extremely rich source of EPA and DHA.

I look at omega-3s as the nutritional building blocks so critical to heart and penis health. For decades, there has been a growing body of evidence supporting fish consumption, and medical researchers have been singing the praises of eating fish as a way to reduce heart attacks by as much as 50 percent.

Scientists have looked closely at the fish-eating cultures of Japan and the Inuits of North America, and they have linked their low rates of cardiovascular disease directly to the EPA/DHA found in the fish they eat. Similarly, the sinking levels of omega-3s in the American diet is most likely related to the rise we have witnessed in heart disease and, yes, erection problems. Scientists reporting in leading medical journals have noted that the higher the intake of EPA/DHA, the lower the likelihood of coronary artery disease and sudden death due to cardiac ailments, as well as a positive effect on asthma and memory issues.

GOOD FAT VS. BAD FAT

If you are wondering how anything openly professing to be "fatty" could possibly be good for your heart and penis, then you need to first understand the difference between the good fats and bad ones. There are four major categories of fat found in the foods we eat: cholesterol, saturated fatty acids, monounsaturated fatty acids, and polyunsaturated fatty acids. The first group, cholesterol, can itself be divided into "good" cholesterol (or high-density lipoproteins) and "bad" cholesterol (low-density lipoproteins). It goes without saying that too much LDL cholesterol can wreak havoc on the arteries by promoting a thick buildup of plaque, which in turn can lead to heart attack, stroke, and yes, diminished hardness. Of the three other categories of fat, only saturated fats, which are found mostly in animal and dairy products, are guilty of raising LDL cholesterol levels.

Omega-3s, however, are polyunsaturated fats, which are actually good for you. In fact, omega-3s are termed "essential fatty acids" because they are so important in promoting good health. Unlike other types of fatty acids, however, the body cannot manufacture omega-3s on its own, and this is the reason why it is so "essential" to make sure you are receiving enough of them from your diet. Most of us do not, and that is a major health concern.

A dramatic shift has taken place over the past one hundred years or so in how the population of this country gets its food. The replacement of seafood, wild greens, and free-range animal meat by processed and fast foods as the mainstays of the average American's diet has led to a marked decrease in the amount of omega-3s that we typically consume.

At the same time, the average dietary level of a similar fatty acid, omega-6, has increased by a remarkable 1,000 percent. This is primarily due to the proliferation of omega-6s in bread, baked goods, and other processed foods as a means of creating longer shelf lives for food products. And while omega-6s are also essential fatty acids and good for you, this huge imbalance between the amounts of omega-3s and omega-6s in the modern diet has literally changed the composition of people's body chemistry.

Omega-6s are similar in molecular composition to omega-3s, and this disparate proportion is thought to create a situation in which the omega-3s may be blocked from getting inside cells to replenish depleted stores in the body.

What people need to do is bring a healthier balance back to their diets. The best way to ensure you consume enough essential omega-3 fatty acids is with daily omega-3 supplementation.

*H*ey, No Fair! He Got Two!

Approximately eighty cases have been reported in medical literature of men born with two penises. A **diphallus** can present as either one organ that separates into two or as two distinct organs. The penises can be side by side, on top of each other, or in separate locations.

*T*hat's Okay, One Will Do

Most men with **diphalluses** are sterile.

GETTING YOUR OMEGA-3S

Omega-3s are found in the highest concentration in fish, particularly salmon, tuna, mackerel, lake trout, and sardines. In order to effectively raise your levels of omega-3s to where you begin to reap the benefits of better penile health, at least two servings of broiled or baked fish a week are necessary. You can also up your dietary dosage by using canola or soybean oil instead of other vegetable oils. Flaxseeds and walnuts are additional sources of omega-3s.

For those of you without the time or inclination to run around harpooning whales like the Inuits, or if you merely lack the discipline or flexibility to eat a steady diet of tuna and salmon, I wholeheartedly recommend omega-3 marine fish oil supplements. With the possible exception of the occasional occurrence of an unpleasant fishy aftertaste, you should experience no side effects. I have found that taking the capsules with orange juice can help to mask the taste, while refrigerating those capsules will also help reduce the incidence of any fishy burps.

THE HARDNESS FACTOR OMEGA-3 PROGRAM

Just how much omega-3 does one need to consume each day for heart, brain, and penis protection? Ideally, your **diet should supply at least 2 g of omega-3s per day.** It is possible to get enough omega-3s from dietary sources but it is very difficult. At least **two fish meals a day** are necessary for cardio and penis protection, which is a lot of fish for most people. Also, many people have a concern about mercury in fish, as well as PCPs, which is why an omega-3 supplement plan makes so much sense.

continued

Omega-3 supplements are available everywhere now. I use the Res-Q 1250 brand from N3 Oceanic, the early pioneer in developing high potency EPA/DHA capsules. In addition, their production plant is located in Norway, where they have an abundant supply of spearing, a cold-water, sardinelike fish that has extremely high levels of EPA/DHA. Another leading brand is Heart Health Essential Omega-3 from Market America. Unlike many other fish oil supplements on the market today, their product provides a science-based, therapeutic dose of three grams of EPA (eicosapentaenoic acid) and DHA (docosahexanoic acid). In addition, their Heart Health System features three powerful formulas, including a daily dose of omega-3. This specially designed supplement combination supports optimal heart health protection utilizing omega-3 fish oils and other vitamins that have been proven to promote a healthy heart.

I have one caveat about omega-3s: Check the amounts of EPA and DHA on the bottle label. I am amazed at the overall poor quality of fish oil capsules found on drugstore and health food store shelves. Many brands of omega-3 capsules do not contain adequate amounts of EPA and DHA to achieve maximum cardiac and penile protection. At **a minimum,** make sure the omega-3 supplement you purchase **contains 400 mg of EPA and 300 mg of DHA.** These highly concentrated capsules will typically cost more than other brands. However, the higher cost is offset by having to take only **2 capsules a day** to achieve the pharmaceutical potency. With a less expensive brand, you may have to take as many as 8 or 10 capsules a day to equal the DHA/EPA found in 2 capsules of the more expensive brand.

I want you to begin by taking **2 g of omega-3 supplements each day,** preferably with a meal.

SEXUAL FITNESS ACTIVITY

You are beginning your third week of the program. If you have been walking daily and achieving your step totals, you have probably noticed that you have lost a few pounds and that your waist size has shrunk a little. That is a good sign because body fat around your middle increases your risk of developing Type 2 diabetes, a primary erection killer. As you pare away this fat, your health profile improves significantly. It goes without saying that you are definitely stronger and more limber, thanks to your daily resistance exercises and stretching. Keep up the good work!

SENSUAL NUTRITION—AS HARD AS YOUR FOOD

Ah, tomatoes. I don't know about you, but when I see a nice big red tomato, all I can think about is getting out my knife, cutting up the red beauty into five or six slices, laying some sliced mozzarella on top, drizzling the combo with heart-healthy extra-virgin Italian olive oil and sprinkling it all with minced fresh basil, a dash of fresh ground pepper, and sea salt. I often fix this summer lunch for myself at the office, and it's enough to carry me through the rest of the afternoon.

The reason I bring up the tomato is because this fruit (yes fruit, since tomatoes develop from flowers and have one or more seeds) is a major source of lycopene, which belongs to a family of nutrients known as carotenoids. Carotenoids are the natural plant pigments found in red, orange, and yellow fruits and vegetables, as well as in green leafy vegetables. Lycopene is a powerful antioxidant that protects tissues, DNA, and other cellular structures from free radicals, the toxic compounds that can harm blood vessels and nerve cells.

For years, researchers have understood the power of lycopene. Scientists have reported that men eating ten or more servings of tomato-based foods per week had a 35 percent reduction in the incidence of prostate cancer compared to men who hardly ate any tomato-based foods. Tomato-based foods include pasta sauce, pizza, barbecue sauce, ketchup, and soup. Research also points to lycopene as a key ingredient in heart disease prevention because it lowers low-density lipoprotein (the "bad" type) through its strong antioxidant action, and inhibits the many enzymes involved in cholesterol production.

A European study of 1,300 men compared body fat concentrations of lycopene (lycopene is stored in fat) in men who had a heart attack with men who had not. The researchers reported that those men whose fat had high concentrations of lycopene had half the heart attack risk as those with low levels of the carotenoid. In a study from Finland, lycopene was seen to play an important possible role in the prevention of atherosclerosis, the lethal buildup of fatty plaque on artery walls, which narrows blood vessels. Those Finns with the lowest lycopene consumption had the most signs of atherosclerosis.

Our bodies cannot produce lycopene or any of the other carotenoids. We depend solely on what we eat in order to maintain the protective levels that we need. Therefore, this week, I want you to go to your local farmer's market, roadside stand, or supermarket and buy some fresh vine-ripened red tomatoes. In addition to lycopene, tomatoes are a good source of vitamins C and A, as well as potassium, folic acid, phytoene (another powerful antioxidant carotenoid), and a variety of other phytonutrients.

Lycopene is a fat-soluble substance, which means that in order to be absorbed through the intestines so it can do its good work, it must be consumed with some fat at the same meal. Monounsaturated olive oil fits the bill here. To really get the most available lycopene, however, the tomatoes need to be cooked (with a little oil), which releases the maximum amount of lycopene from its fibrous cell walls. If you happen to like tomato juice, make sure it is made from cooked tomatoes to get the most powerful benefits.

⦿ QUICK TOMATO SAUCE

So simple, so good. Make your quick tomato sauce for pasta, rice, fish, or meat in a large, heavy saucepan.

¼ cup olive oil
1 clove garlic, minced
3–4 fresh tomatoes (or 1 28-oz. can whole tomatoes)
1 teaspoon coarse sea salt or kosher salt, plus more to taste
1 teaspoon black pepper, plus more to taste
1 teaspoon fresh basil, chopped

1. Heat olive oil over medium heat.
2. When olive oil is hot, sauté garlic for 5 minutes. Be careful not to burn garlic.
3. Wash tomatoes and remove stems.
4. Dice the tomatoes and add to olive oil.
5. Simmer over medium heat for 10 to 15 minutes, stirring periodically, until tomatoes wilt and are lightly cooked.
6. Add salt, pepper, and basil to taste.
7. The sauce can be cooled and stored in the refrigerator for up to one week or frozen up to three months.

Try the following recipes from Waldy this week

⦿ MENU ONE

TURKEY PAILLARDS WITH BLACK PEPPER, SAGE, AND GARLIC

Spicy Potato Salad with Sweet and Hot Peppers
Turkey Paillards with Black Pepper, Sage, and Garlic
Grilled Pineapple with Gin, Juniper, and Lime

⦿ MENU TWO

HALIBUT WITH LEMON CONFIT AND WHITE WINE

Seared Filet Mignon Tartare
Halibut with Lemon Confit and White Wine
Individual Warm Chocolate Cake with Roasted Apricots
(See **Appendix II** for recipes)

WEEK FOUR   WEEK FIVE   WEEK SIX

HALFWAY THROUGH—CELEBRATE WITH A COMPANION

Congratulations are certainly in order this week: You are passing the halfway mark of the program and by now you are definitely experiencing many positive changes in how you look and feel. You should be proud of yourself and your accomplishments. I applaud your efforts at taking control of your health!

To really make your body work for you later—whether that's a "quickie" 100-meter dash or a longer love-fest marathon—feed it right. Remember that dinner is not the main event, but only fuel for the fire. Ensuring that you meet your basic needs will enhance your performance. Prepare a sensuous dinner at home with your partner or else go out to a favorite restaurant. Whatever your choice, keep these nutritional guidelines in mind:

HALFWAY MILESTONE DINNER

PEPPERED TUNA WITH RED WINE AND SHALLOTS

Chilled Yellow Tomato Soup
Peppered Tuna with Red Wine and Shallots
Peaches with Balsamic Vinegar and Roquefort
Green Tea
(See **Appendix II** for recipes)

Dining Out Option

For those of you who want to go out—and why not for a change?—there are several important guidelines I want you to adhere to in order to make this a very special occasion:

▶ This special evening is all a matter of perception. It is not about you having sex tonight but rather it's about you feeling confident that if the occasion arises, you will be able to perform, without a second thought.

▶ Reduce and eliminate all possible stressors; don't leave anything to chance.

- Choose a familiar restaurant. Make the reservations well in advance.

- Do not go to an "all you can eat" restaurant.

- Take a pass on all high-fat foods. This includes fried, basted, braised, au gratin, escalloped, sautéed, and creamy selections.

- Make your choice from the steamed, broiled, baked, grilled, poached, or roasted dishes.

- Skip all foods high in salt or MSG, as well as gravy and sauces.

- When choosing salad dressing, ask that it be served on the side.

- If you order red meat, trim the fat. Have poultry served without skin.

- To keep portion size down, split your entrée with your partner or order appetizer portions instead.

- For dessert, choose fruit or sherbet.

- Don't overeat. Bring leftovers home.

- Make sure that you don't drink too much. Every sip you take ultimately has an impact on your sexual chemistry.

- Focus on your partner at dinner. Don't start thinking about after dinner—stay in the here and now.

ANOTHER GUY THING—FEAR OF DOCTORS

After more than thirty years of medical practice, I have concluded that many men are afraid of doctors. They look upon going to a physician as some undesirable form of pampering, no matter how sick they are. In general, men are not all that good at taking care of their health, probably because they have not grown up with periodic medical exams. Women, on the other hand, are comfortable with routine exams for gynecological checkups and pregnancy. And since women also tend to be the family caregiver, making health-care decisions for children and taking them to the doctor has typically been a mother's role.

Code Red

A man goes to the doctor one day and says, "Doc, I have a problem. My penis is red."

The doctor says, "Drop your pants and let me take a look." So the man does.

"No problem," says the doctor. "We can have you fixed up in no time. That'll be $40."

The man's so impressed that he tells a friend about the experience and that he hadn't been to a doctor who charged only $40 in ages.

"What doctor did you go to?" his friend says. "I have a similar problem."

So a few days later, his friend goes to the same doctor and tells him, "Doc, you've got to help me. My penis is blue."

The doctor asks to take a look. "Ah yes . . . Ummm . . . Yep, we can take care of it, no problem. $400."

"FOUR HUNDRED DOLLARS? Wait a minute! You took care of my friend for only $40."

"Yes, I did," says the doctor. "But his penis had lipstick on it. Yours has gangrene!"

The typical man will go for years without ever seeing a doctor. They are not trained to think about early detection of disease. If men do not have any symptoms, they tend to think they are fine, so understandably it is hard to convince them to go in for basic screening tests for cholesterol, colon and prostate cancer, glaucoma, and diabetes. Also, when symptoms of an ailment do occur, men will oftentimes ignore or underestimate them. They do their best to tough it out, often allowing a minor problem to escalate into something more risky before they finally consent to see a doctor.

Unfortunately, this traditional masculine pattern can be hazardous not only to their health, but to the health of their partner. Here's how:

▶ Untreated hardness problems, often a sign of underlying heart disease, hypertension, or diabetes, can make sex difficult, if not impossible, and can quickly strain it to the breaking point.

▶ Sleep apnea, with its nocturnal snoring and lapses in breathing, is not only harmful to the man, but will disrupt a partner's sleep, leaving them sleep deprived and unable to function during the day.

▶ Untreated or poorly managed depression can rip a relationship apart with its incapacitating profile of absence of joy and inability to function at work.

▶ Excessive drinking, drug abuse as a result of stress, and untreated hypertension are all ailments that can trigger enough stress to cause a decline in the partner's health.

If this sounds at all like you, here is what I want you to do this week. Communication is vital and an open and honest discussion is warranted with your partner. Explain that you now understand that your health is in fact your responsibility. I want you to promise that you will take care of your own health. Then follow through.

Since this is a relationship of equals, explain that you want to make this a true partnership, and that you want to be healthy together. Decide together on your health goals for the coming months and write them down. Figure out together how you will achieve them. An annual checkup with your doctor is a good starting point. Let your doctor determine what your health profile indicates and follow through with suggestions for improvement.

THE BLUES CAN BE A MEDICAL CONDITION

Depression affects about 6 million American men annually. While many people often link depression with psychological distress and pain, feeling "blue," and having constant thoughts of worthlessness, mental health experts are now noticing that some physical complaints are tip-offs to an underlying depression.

The exact causes of depression are unclear. Current psychiatric thinking is that certain biochemical imbalances in the brain ultimately lead to depression, possibly stemming from a defect in the communication between neurons (nerve cells) in the brain. Chemical changes occur in the brain during depression, and researchers believe that these changes produce the symptoms of depression.

Unfortunately, many people simply don't know what depression is, or they think that they can overcome it with sheer willpower. They cannot. It's now estimated that 15 percent of all chronic cases of depression end in suicide, with men taking their lives on average four times more often than women.

One recent study of more than 1,000 people who were eventually diagnosed with depression reported that physical symptoms were either the only complaint or a major complaint in almost 70 percent of the subjects.

> **Yes, Sometimes It Is All in Your Mind**
>
> Changes and significant fluctuations in erection hardness can be the first sign of an underlying physical or psychiatric condition. It can be a physical manifestation of depression—talk to your doctor.

MEDICATIONS TO THE RESCUE

One major approach for treating depression is with antidepressant medications. There are several advantages of treating depression with medication: The drugs are effective against mild, moderate, and severe forms of major depression. Patients usually respond more quickly to drugs than psychotherapy (as much as two weeks sooner). They are easy to administer. In addition, the medications are not addictive, and, when properly administered, are rarely dangerous.

For some men, depression can cause hardness problems or a significant loss of interest in sex. For others, however, hardness problems themselves—whether caused by high blood pressure, diabetes, elevated cholesterol, or specific medications to treat these ailments—can actually cause mild depression. When popular antidepressant medications are added to the mix, as good as they are, they can often negatively affect hardness and overall sexual function.

Those medications that affect the vascular system—including blood pressure, the heart, and the respiratory organs—will have an impact on any blood-delivering system in the body. Some hamper the blood vessels in the penis by constricting them, thereby making it virtually impossible to achieve an erection. Others affect the nerves that activate penile responsiveness. Then there are the medications that strike

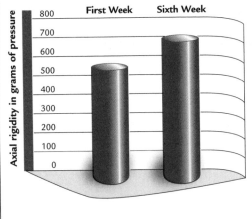

HARDNESS FACTOR 6 WEEKS
Depressed and Soft

Taking daily medication for his depression for the first time, the 42-year-old executive saw his sex drive diminish along with his hardness. Low DIR readings of 525 and 600 (**DIR Avg. 562**) were not surprising, considering his previous mental state. After agreeing to complete the Six-Week Program, he was happy to see a boost in his outlook as well as a 25 percent jump in his DIR readings (**DIR Avg. 702**). The regular exercise—which made him feel better—and increased hardness encouraged him to repeat another six-week session to help increase his hardness and overall health.

Axial rigidity in grams of pressure

First Week   Sixth Week

800
700
600
500
400
300
200
100
0

Patient #28 • 42 years old

the areas of the brain where desire and sexual pleasure are centered, resulting in a severe decrease in sex drive.

If you suddenly notice that you are having erection problems where none existed before, take a good look at any—and all—medications that you are currently using. Bring this up with your doctor. When the lines of communication between you and your doctor are kept open, it is usually possible to change or adjust medication. The goal is to maintain your general health while not adversely affecting your hardness and sexual performance.

Not Tonight, Dear, I Have a Migraine

CHUCK, age 36 —The beta male

Chuck was a new patient with an old complaint. He had been having regular sex with his partner, a fellow actor, for more than a month but recently found that he couldn't get a hard erection anymore. "Everything was great with Tony until it came to sex. He wanted me and was always hard when we started fooling around. I was too but then I would start to soften; he took this as a lack of sexual interest. It was after a few more softies that he broke off the relationship. That's why I'm here to see you."

After going over the medications he was taking, Chuck mentioned he had recently been prescribed a beta blocker by another physician to relieve his persistent migraine headaches. A beta blocker is a medicine that's generally used to treat high blood pressure and heart problems, but it's also effective for migraine treatment as well. Since the drug blocks the influence of stress hormones on the heart, reducing blood pressure and heart rate, a side effect of the drug is decreased hardness.

Two weeks later, after switching Chuck to a different migraine medication, he told me that his hardness problems had completely cleared up. Tony was also back in his life, and he had just won a part in a new TV sitcom. "Life couldn't be better," he said.

DEPRESSION CHECKLIST

Every year more than 18 million Americans suffer from clinical depression. Clinical depression often goes untreated because people fail to recognize its many symptoms.

Check off any symptoms of clinical depression you may be experiencing:

1. Do you feel a persistent sad, anxious, or empty mood?
   ○ **Yes**   ○ **No**

2. Are you sleeping too little or sleeping too much?
   ○ **Yes**   ○ **No**

3. Do you have a reduced appetite and weight loss or increased appetite and weight gain?
   ○ **Yes**   ○ **No**

4. Are you experiencing a decrease in sex drive (libido)?
   ○ **Yes**   ○ **No**

5. Have you noticed a loss of interest or pleasure in activities once enjoyed?
   ○ **Yes**   ○ **No**

6. Are you restless or irritable?
   ○ **Yes**   ○ **No**

7. Do you suffer from persistent physical symptoms that do not respond to treatment, such as headaches, chronic pain, or constipation and other digestive disorders?
   ○ **Yes**   ○ **No**

8. Have you noticed difficulty concentrating, remembering, or making decisions?
   ○ **Yes**   ○ **No**

9. Are you feeling constant fatigue or loss of energy?
   ○ **Yes**   ○ **No**

10. Is there a sense of feeling guilty, hopeless, or worthless?
    ○ **Yes**   ○ **No**

11. Are you having thoughts of death or suicide?
    ○ **Yes**   ○ **No**

NOTE: If you experience five or more of these symptoms for longer than two weeks, or if the symptoms are severe enough to interfere with your daily routines, see your doctor or a qualified mental health professional. The good news is that almost everyone who is treated can soon feel better.

> ### HEADACHE LESSONS
>
> **Lesson 1**   A variety of prescription drugs can both increase and decrease sexual interest and performance.
>
> **Lesson 2**   Erections require the orchestration of nerves, blood vessels, and hormones, and many drugs and herbal stimulants affect this process.

TAKING CARE OF YOUR PROSTATE

Prostate cancer is the most common cancer in men, and, following lung cancer, the major cause of cancer death among American men. The likelihood of developing prostate cancer increases with age. The lifetime risk for prostate cancer is 1 out of every 6 American men, with 1 of 30 dying from the disease. For still unknown reasons, the incidence of mortality from prostate cancer is higher among African American men.

But because this disease is such a slow-growing ailment, most men are more likely to die *with* prostate cancer than they are *from* it. Once a man has prostate cancer, he has about a 3 percent risk of dying from it.

The prostate is the walnut-sized organ located at the base of the bladder. The prostate supplies some of the fluids in the ejaculation, which is the semen that supports the sperm. This is required to give sperm an energy source, as well as a proper environment until it fertilizes the egg.

At birth, the prostate is the size of a pea and reaches normal size by age 20. When a man turns 40, the prostate often begins to grow. When the prostate grows it can do one of three things: it can swell and grow and give no symptoms at all; grow and compress the urethra, the tube running from the bladder through the prostate, where the urine flows through, creating symptoms of blockage; or it can grow and become cancerous. Once prostate cancer develops, it usually grows slowly over many years. Only rarely does it grow and spread rapidly.

Each year an estimated 189,000 new cases of prostate cancer are diagnosed in the United States. Unfortunately, 30,000 are expected to die of the disease. A positive prostate cancer diagnosis can certainly be a shock but thanks to early detection with routine PSA (prostate-specific antigen) testing, most men are now diagnosed with disease confined to the prostate gland, where it is curable. The good news is that local therapies—surgery to remove the gland or radiation—are better than ever.

A man should have his first PSA test at age 40, using a PSA cutoff point of 4.0 nanograms per milliliter (ng/ml) of blood. Although a reading of 4 ng/ml has been traditionally accepted as an indication of the possibility of prostate cancer, there is now a progressive group of urologic researchers who recommend a PSA cutoff of 2.5 ng/ml at age 40. If a man has an initial PSA above 2.5 ng/ml, the doctor should be on alert for a possible cancer. If a man is below that 2.5 ng/ml mark, he will have his next PSA test when he is 45, followed by another when he is 50. PSA tests are then performed every other year until he reaches 70. The man will then complete a very extensive personal history, documenting not only his PSA scores, but his PSA velocity, a marker of how quickly a man's PSA level goes up over time.

> ***H**ow're They Hangin'?*
>
> The left testicle usually hangs lower than the right for right-handers, while the opposite is true for lefties.

DON'T LET IT GO TO YOUR HEAD

Benign prostatic hyperplasia, or BPH, a noncancerous enlargement of the prostate gland, is a common part of the aging process for many men. BPH can cause the gland to compress the urethra, making urination difficult, painful, or both.

The popular drug finasteride (Proscar, Propecia), which is designed for treating BPH and male pattern baldness, works by inhibiting an enzyme that triggers the conversion of testosterone to dihydrotestosterone, the most potent androgen inside the prostate cells. In the prostate, reduction of androgen reduces the volume of the prostate and can improve urinary flow in the process. The drug can shrink the prostate by as much as 30 percent by interfering with the hormonal chain of events that maintain prostate volume.

One caveat: Finasteride has its own limitations. It takes three to six months to work, must be used daily, and has only moderate ability to improve symptoms. Some men may also find that their ejaculatory volumes are reduced, and a small percentage report sexual dysfunction with long-term use of the drug. These side effects, however, disappear when the drug is discontinued.

Also, since finasteride lowers PSA levels by 50 percent after six months of treatment, in order to best assess prostate cancer risk, the PSA value must be multiplied by 2 to achieve an accurate reading. It's imperative that you alert your doctor that you are using this drug if he wasn't the physician who started you on the treatment to get accurate test readings. A full head of hair is nice, prostate cancer is not.

> ### *T*he Ball's in Your Court
>
> The word *testis* comes from the Latin, meaning "witness," and shares the same root with "testify." Some speculate that the modern term, *testicles*, derives from the ancient Roman practice of a man's bearing witness or "testifying" by holding his testes as he spoke.

Self-Examination: Because You Can

ALEX, age 21—A lump in his throat

Alex feared the worst. The 21-year-old college senior had felt a hard lump on his testicle. His thoughts turned to testicular cancer, which is why he had come to see me, his hair still damp from his shower.

Lance Armstrong, the six-time Tour de France winner, had

testicular cancer and beat it. To date, his popular sunny yellow "LIVESTRONG" wristbands have been among the hottest accessories, helping raise millions of dollars for cancer research. Alex, a recreational cyclist, had one on his right wrist in memory of his father who had died from prostate cancer.

Most men know nothing about testicular cancer. Armstrong ignored the cancer's warning signs in 1996, and it later spread to his abdomen, lungs, and brain. Even fewer men know how they can detect it themselves. Testicular cancer is rare, accounting for just 1 percent of all cancers. Although it can strike at any age, the prime years are between 15 and 25, with white males at the highest risk. Each year there are close to 7,000 cases and more than 300 deaths. However, when detected early enough, the survival rate approaches 100 percent.

Although there is no way to prevent testicular cancer, a regular monthly three-minute self-exam, like the monthly breast self-exam for women, is the best way to detect this cancer in its earliest stages.

After a warm bath or shower, which relaxes the scrotal skin, gently roll each testicle between the thumb and forefinger of both hands. A normal testis moves freely within the scrotum. It is also normal for one testicle to be larger than the other. Both should be smooth and firm. See if there is any change from the way it feels normally. Contact your physician immediately if you feel any hard lumps, nodules, or swelling.

Testicular cancer begins in one or both of the testicles. Symptoms of testicular cancer include a slight enlargement of one of the testes and a change in its consistency. There may be no localized pain, but often there is a dull ache in the lower abdomen and groin area. The preferred treatment for testicular cancer is surgical removal of the affected testicle.

Luckily for Alex, the slight swelling in his testicle was from a varicocele, a mass of enlarged veins that lead from the testicle.

What's Shakin', Mate?

When men of Australia's Walibri tribe greet each other, they shake penises instead of hands.

A varicocele can develop in one testicle or both, but is typically found on the left side. The cause is often a defective valve that normally allows blood to flow from the testicle toward the abdomen. These enlarged veins are very common and are present in 15 percent of men. Varicoceles may be responsible for low sperm counts and can affect fertility. Since the varicocele did not cause Alex any testicular pain or discomfort and he wasn't planning to start a family, I told him he wouldn't need any surgical repair at this time.

SIX-WEEK PROGRAM

1. HARDNESS FACTOR

Rate your current level of hardness for Day Twenty-one of the program. (Check off one box.)

○ Soft   ○ Soft/Hard   ○ Hard
○ Very Hard   ○ Like a Steel Beam

2. SEXUAL FITNESS

FROM WEEKS 1–2:
- The Side Lunge Reach (10 repetitions)
- Angry Cat Stretch (3 times)

1. The Woodchopper Exercise NEW

The Woodchopper is a total body warm-up for the muscles of the upper and lower body, including the chest, back, shoulders, core, and legs.

- Stand with your feet shoulder-width apart, raise your arms up, stretching toward the ceiling with your abdominals drawn in toward your spine.
- Bend your knees while keeping your chest lifted and swing both of your arms between your legs as if you were chopping wood.
- Repeat 10 times.
- Classic Push-Ups (3 sets of 8 reps) or Modified Push-Ups (3 sets of 10 reps)
- Plank (3 sets, hold 45 seconds, rest 15 seconds)
- Cobra (10 repetitions)

2. The Squat NEW

The Squat will strengthen the buttocks, hamstrings, and quadriceps.

- Stand with your arms fully extended in front of you at shoulder height and your feet hip-width apart.
- Keep your back straight and your weight evenly distributed over both your feet.
- Slowly squat down as if you were going to sit in a chair, lowering yourself until the tops of your thighs are parallel to the floor.
- Pause for 1 second.
- Slowly rise to standing position.
- Repeat 10 times.

3. WALKING

Take 7,000 steps a day. Circle each day you achieved this goal:

Sunday Monday Tuesday Wednesday
Thursday Friday Saturday

4. HARDNESS FACTOR SUPPLEMENTS

Take Pycnogenol (80 mg)/L-arginine (3 g) mixture or Pycnogenol Plus or Prelox Blue daily.

Horny Goat Weed (2 500-mg capsules)
Take 2 horny goat weed capsules daily. Take 4 capsules one to two hours prior to a sexual encounter.

Omega-3 Fatty Acids NEW
Take 2 omega-3 capsules daily. Each capsule should contain at least 400 mg of EPA and 300 mg of DHA.

WEEK ONE   WEEK TWO   WEEK THREE

5. SENSUAL NUTRITION

Tomatoes:

Vine-ripened tomatoes drizzled with olive oil can boost lycopene intake and antioxidant protection, both of which can guard against hardness failure. Did you have your "red medicine" this week?

○ **Yes**   ○ **No**

Prepare three sensuous meals this week.

Turkey breast is the leanest of all meats, making it great for health, heart, and hardness. An excellent source of B vitamins, protein, and selenium, each 3-ounce serving of turkey has less than half a gram of fat and barely 120 calories.

Halibut, like other popular lean fish, is low in fat and calories, but rich in high-quality protein. A great alternative to red meat, halibut is an excellent source of omega-3 fatty acids and vitamin E, both of which play a leading role in heart disease prevention.

▶ Turkey Paillards with Black Pepper, Sage, and Garlic
▶ Halibut with Lemon Confit and White Wine
▶ Peppered Tuna with Red Wine and Shallots

A MAN @ 35

Mature sexually and performing at a very high level.

Possesses a better sense of his maleness.

Hardness levels are still high in healthy men, and extremely high in men who practice good health habits.

Men who have not been preserving their health are starting to show clear signs of decline in hardness.

Poor lifestyle choices are starting to impact health with sleep apnea, diabetes, overweight, and hypertension affecting hardness.

THE PENIS & THE PROTRACTOR

120–100 degrees

Head
180 degrees

Feet
0 degrees

DEGREES OF AGE

THE THIRD WEEK—HARDER WE GO

Congratulations are in order. You have finished the first half of the program. Your goals and motivations have changed during the past twenty-one days, which is great. Here are a few questions you need to ask yourself daily: *How do I feel? Am I making the progress I should be making? Am I increasing my hardness?* After taking stock of where you are and where you want to go, find ways to make sure that you meet your personal goals.

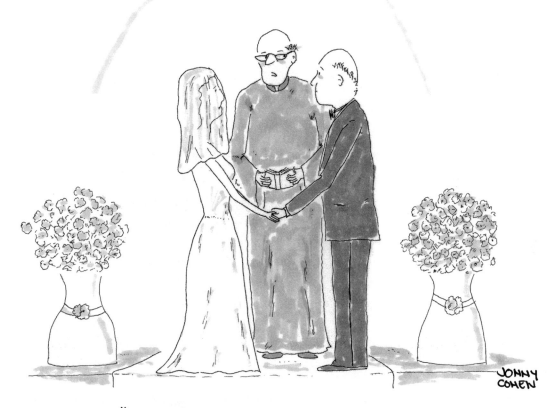

"TIL DEATH OR DYSFUNCTION DO YOU PART?"

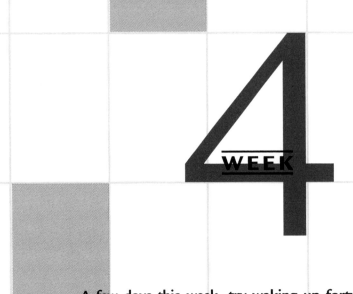

4

WEEK

A few days this week, try waking up forty-five minutes earlier than usual and going for a walk with a friend or your partner. Keep going to bed at 10:30 and this new earlier time won't be an issue. For those of you who have already made great progress with the sexual fitness exercises, try to increase your repetitions to the 10 to 15 range for each exercise. Don't forget to take your supplements. I keep mine on the kitchen table so I'm always reminded.

GETTING HARDER

Reaffirming your commitment to building a healthier, stronger, harder body is one of the best things you can do for yourself. As you move into the second half of the program, find ways to own the program and really incorporate it into your new way of living a happy, healthy, and harder life.

COMING TO GRIPS WITH HARD ISSUES

It's amazing what Viagra did to help bring male sexual issues out of the closet. Years ago, STDs (sexually transmitted diseases) were about the only penis-related topic a man would discuss with his doctor. And that was only because he desperately needed a prescription for penicillin. All that has changed, which is great for men.

Few of us view advertising as a positive social force, but thanks to the multimillion-dollar direct-to-consumer advertising campaigns for erection drugs, some of the embarrassment in discussing hardness disappointments has been taken away. Men are now becoming more comfortable in discussing other personal hardness issues with their physicians, such as premature ejaculation. I welcome this new and open era.

The Fourth-Week Assignments

Sexual Fitness

▶ Increase walking to 8,000 steps a day this week. As your strength and endurance increase entering the Fourth Week of the program, pick up your walking pace a bit. You are also going to work on strengthening your core muscles with the Bridge and augment core stability, upper body strength, and lower body flexibility with the Squat Thrust exercise. Each of these exercises will pay off in the bedroom.

Hardness Factor Supplements

▶ Continue with all the supplements from the previous weeks. This week, I want you to add 200 mg of red wine extract and 100 mg of grape seed extract to your supplement program. Both are excellent sources of oligomeric proanthocyanidins, or OPCs, and will help improve blood flow.

Sensual Nutrition

▶ Change your mindset. Get rid of the notion that certain foods are either "good" or "bad." Once you come to see all foods as types of fuel for your daily activities, your eating habits will change for the better.
▶ Blueberries are antioxidant powerhouses. Look for wild blueberries from Maine or Canada at your local farm stand, or pick up a few boxes of cultivated berries at your supermarket this week. When blueberries are plentiful and less expensive at the market, pick up an extra box and put it in the freezer. To defrost, put a serving in a colander under running water. You'll have fresh berries all year long!

HARDNESS FACTOR SUPPLEMENTS— STICKS AND STEMS

This week I want you to start taking two other oligomeric proantho-cyanidins (OPCs). These are two additional turbocharged members of the flavonoid family. You are already taking OPCs and did not realize it. In Week One, you started by taking Pycnogenol, a supplement made from the bark of the French maritime pine tree. In Week Two, I asked that you start drinking black or green tea. I want you to now add red wine extract and grape seed extract to your supplement list to boost your penis and heart protection.

What I like so much about the OPCs is their potent antioxidant impact on free radicals within the body. As you will recall, free radicals are molecules or atoms with a free electron, which makes them react easily with other molecules. Supplementation with OPCs helps neutralize these cell-damaging compounds in the body.

VOILÀ! THE "FRENCH PARADOX"

There is a growing body of evidence linking red wine consumption with a reduced risk of cardiovascular disease. Scientists now believe that resveratrol—the OPC compound found in the skin of the red grape, and in grape seed itself—is responsible for the enhanced heart protection.

These two OPCs might also explain the so-called "French paradox." Consumers of high-fat foods (butter, cream, eggs, cheese, and foie gras, just to name a few), and often heavy-duty smokers, the French nonetheless do not have the problem with heart disease that is rampant in the United States.

In France, the typical person still outlives his or her American counterpart by about 2.5 years (76.5 versus 74 years). More impressive, however, is that in spite of French lifestyle behaviors, they nevertheless suffer 40 percent fewer heart attacks than Americans. Hence, the paradox.

WEEK FOUR *WEEK FIVE* *WEEK SIX*

REACH FOR THE SUPPLEMENTS, NOT THE WINE

Red wine is an excellent source of resveratrol but the problem with adopting the French custom of drinking red wine with lunch and dinner to ward off heart disease is that it encourages alcohol consumption. The concern with alcohol consumption is both the danger of addiction and abuse along with the more prosaic caloric impact. And even the most health-conscious eater doesn't get the full benefits of a balanced diet—which, of course, includes the proper amount of fruits and vegetables. Foods lose much of their antioxidant powers once they are frozen, processed, or cooked. This is why I want you to supplement your diet this week with both red wine extract and grape seed extract.

RED WINE EXTRACT FOR THE HEART AND HARDNESS

Grapes produce resveratrol naturally as a fungicide to protect the plant against mildew that is common in some cool, humid, wine-growing regions. Researchers believe that resveratrol is partially responsible for the cholesterol-lowering effects of wine.

Recent studies suggest that by inhibiting fat deposits in the blood vessels, the antioxidant properties of resveratrol may result in reduced risk of cardiovascular disease, lowered total cholesterol, and lowered LDL cholesterol.

PICKING GRAPE SEED EXTRACT

Just as its name implies, grape seed extract comes from the seeds of the red grapes typically used to make wine. These seeds are rich in OPCs and will help improve blood circulation by preventing the development of harmful plaque that can obstruct arteries.

Grape seeds are so potent because they contain three types of flavonoids. Catechins are notable for their ability to help stave off the effects of atherosclerosis, the hardening of the arteries. When the arteries harden, there is no way you can get a good erection.

In addition to the catechins, oligomers in the grape seeds help lower blood pressure, while polymers act as good all-around free-radical battlers. These three flavonoids work together to keep your penile vessels clear of plaque and functioning optimally.

THE HARDNESS FACTOR **OPC PROGRAM**

The **daily recommendation** for antioxidant-rich fruits and vegetables is **five to nine servings.** I know most of my patients don't even come close to eating this much, which is why I recommend OPCs—like **Pycnogenol, red wine extract,** and **grape seed extract**—to all of my patients. The grape seed flavonoids help thwart damage to the lining of the blood vessels by protecting the elastin and collagen that make up the vessels. This helps ensure a steady supply of oxygen and other nutrients to the heart, brain, and penis.

Take **100 mg of grape seed extract (300 mg if you are a smoker) and 25 mg of red wine extract daily.** When taken in combination with **vitamins E and C,** which you will start in **Week Five,** the OPCs enhance the **effectiveness** of **vitamin E by 50 times** and **vitamin C by 20 times.** That's an antioxidant force that will certainly offer the most free-radical protection possible.

I use Isotonix OPC-3, a natural food supplement made up of a combination of grape seed, red wine, and pine bark extracts. Mixed with water to form an isotonic solution to supply the body's chemical needs, it is well absorbed in the lower intestine within five minutes.

NOTE: Check the Hardness Factor Shopping List **(page 327)** for recommended OPC choices.

WEEK FOUR   *WEEK FIVE*   *WEEK SIX*

SENSUAL NUTRITION

Whenever you wonder what snack food will taste great and provide a healthy antioxidant wallop, think blueberries. Those tiny blue nutrition superstars contain more disease-fighting, heart-protecting antioxidants than just about any other fruit or vegetable. In addition, their unique tanginess and sweetness will have you polishing off a box with no problem.

Blueberries derive their power from anthocyanins, a separate class of flavonoids from OPCs. Anthocyanins are naturally-occurring compounds that impart color to fruit, vegetables, and plants and are thought to play a major role with their high antioxidant activity. Close to three hundred anthocyanins have been discovered.

By following the Hardness Factor Program and maximizing hardness, you also maximize your heart protection:

- Eat 5-9 servings of fruits and vegetables daily: heart attack risk drops 30 percent.
- Engage in physical activity daily (walk 10,000 steps): heart attack risk drops 14 percent.
- Limit alcohol to 0-2 drinks daily: heart attack risk drops 9 percent.

ERECTION Rx

Nothing says "Game Over" to a sexual encounter more than premature ejaculation (PE), a problem that affects 25 percent of men on a regular basis. So great is the embarrassment of climaxing too soon that this little-discussed yet very common male bedroom problem is the one men are least likely to talk about with anyone.

The widespread incidence of premature ejaculation suggests that it is probably encoded deep in our genetic makeup as some sort of survival benefit. When we were still living in caves or out under the stars, we were easy prey when sexually aroused. Approaching orgasm, a man was aware of nothing around him but the sensations in his penis. Climaxing quickly may not have satisfied his partner, but it kept him out of the clutches of wild animals and enemies. While quick shooters may not have changed much over the millennia, we do have the ability to delay, to slow down the inevitable. It's now estimated that anywhere from 20 to 30 percent of American men have PE, which is defined as a persistent or recurrent ejaculation with minimal sexual stimulation before, upon, or shortly after penetration, or before the person wishes to ejaculate.

PE is oftentimes a matter of perspective. The typical man takes between five and ten minutes to reach orgasm. If a man's partner reaches orgasm in five minutes and the man in seven, leaving both completely satisfied, this is not PE. However, if a man lasts fifteen minutes before climaxing and losing his hard erection, but his partner needs twenty minutes to reach orgasm, then it could be considered PE. It all depends on each person's point of view.

This week I want you to work on increasing your staying power. You and your partner will be very happy with the results.

Check the Expiration Date

A healthy male manufactures several hundred million sperm each day, which are then stored. The sperm a man emits today was actually produced more than three weeks ago.

Over Before It Begins: Premature Ejaculation

RICK, age 28—"The minuteman"

As part of her periodic physical exam, I asked Joanne if she was satisfied with her sex life. The vibrant 28-year-old Manhattan real estate agent didn't skip a beat: "No, I'm not satisfied," she said. "But it has nothing to do with me. It's my new boyfriend, Rick. He's got premature ejaculation. I call him my minuteman. With Rick, intercourse is typically all finished in less than sixty seconds."

I told Joanne that premature ejaculation, or PE, is by far the most common and underestimated male erection difficulty. The problem is compounded by the fact that men are reluctant to speak about it. However, there are solutions and I suggested that she determine whether Rick would like to pursue a course of treatment.

When Rick came to see me the following week, he acknowledged that PE had been a lifelong problem. He was never able to last longer than thirty seconds after entering a woman's vagina, and there were times when he had actually ejaculated before penetration. "I felt like crawling into a hole and disappearing after that happened," he said. "Women are very disappointed, to say the least. Some have even become angry with me."

> 66 Just as some men need antihistamines for allergies for the rest of their lives, so too will some men need lifelong medication to delay their orgasms.

There are now several oral medications that are being used by men with PE, I told Rick. What I frequently offer patients with PE is a trial run with 50 mg of Zoloft, a very low dose of a popular SSRI antidepressant. When used off-label like this and taken four hours before a sexual encounter, the drug effectively delays orgasm.

Some of my patients who have used antidepressants for PE have found that ejaculation is delayed for as long as five minutes. In addition, with confidence restored and orgasms delayed for much longer periods, some men no longer need medication after a few weeks. There has been a retraining—a different behavior pattern is established. This is not the case for everyone, however. Just as some men need antihistamines for allergies for the rest of their lives, so too will some men need lifelong medication to delay their orgasms.

I reminded Rick that the most important aspect of an intimate relationship is communication. I urged him to talk to Joanne about his PE and try to come up with a mutual solution. I suggested that they both continue to keep an open dialog in the interest of their relationship, thereby removing the additional stress that comes from trying to cope with PE alone. If they were so inclined, the couple could also explore non-pharmacological approaches to PE, including Tantric sex.

<table>
<tr><td colspan="2" align="center">**TIMING LESSONS**</td></tr>
<tr><td>**Lesson 1**</td><td>PE is one of the most common complaints of men and their partners.</td></tr>
<tr><td>**Lesson 2**</td><td>PE can affect men of all ages.</td></tr>
<tr><td>**Lesson 3**</td><td>The causes of PE range from anxiety to sexual inexperience to erectile dysfunction.</td></tr>
<tr><td>**Lesson 4**</td><td>PE may be short-lived or a lifelong problem.</td></tr>
<tr><td>**Lesson 5**</td><td>PE usually can be effectively treated once the exact cause is understood.</td></tr>
</table>

ERECTION DRUGS HELP OVERCOME PE

Another solution for PE, especially for men who have erectile dysfunction, is to take a low dose of Levitra or Viagra before a sexual encounter. Granted, these erection medications help trigger erections with less stimulation, but more importantly for men with PE, they dramatically reduce the refractory period, the time between erections. If a man comes fast with his first erection, he should be able to get a second erection very quickly—thanks to the drug—and last considerably longer as the lovemaking session continues.

THE UNQUICKIE—TANTRIC SEX

The polar opposite of the quickie, this discipline from India removes orgasm as the immediate goal, delaying it for quite some time as the lovers pursue a heightened mind/body sensual experience. The Tantric belief is that our sexual urgings spring from an internal furnace that provides each of us with a vital flow of energy. Reaching climax means sexual energy is lost. But by taking control of sexual desires and putting the brakes on orgasm for

One Final PE Solution

A guy runs into his ex-girlfriend at a bar.

"I had sex with another woman last night," he tells her. "But I was thinking of you the whole time."

"You miss me that much?" she asks.

"No," he says. "But it kept me from coming too fast."

as long as possible, the thinking is, we are able not only to intensify the sexual experience, but to expand our consciousness as we learn new things about ourselves and our partners.

Sexual encounters are long, languid, and sensual. The naked Tantric partners receive enjoyment from lovingly touching and being touched in the same manner as they look into each other's eyes, breathing together in tandem. By focusing on sensations and how they feel about their partner, men are taught to delay orgasm for as long as possible. In the process, lovemaking is stretched to record time and partners become more "connected," intimately bound to each other and the movements of the universe. Besides that the sex is good.

Sometimes a Bed Is for Sleeping

ZACK, age 25—The too-late shift

Zack recently started graduate school and to make ends meet he took a job as a bartender on the late shift at a local gay bar downtown, oftentimes returning home at 2 or 3 in the morning. Getting to his morning classes and keeping up with his studies was difficult, but what was more perplexing to Zack was his sudden difficulty in achieving an erection. "This shouldn't be happening to me. I am only 25 years old," he told me. Frank, his longtime partner, initially thought Zack was having an affair, but soon came to believe there was something medically wrong and had recommended that he come to see me.

"I don't have any interest in other men," he said. "I'm crazy about Frankie. I finally convinced him of that. We are both worried, though. What's wrong with me? Most of the time I just can't get hard, or if I do, it doesn't last very long."

Zack was slim and had a dark tattoo that snaked up his right forearm. It seemed to complement his blood-shot eyes and the dark bags he had under his eyes. "How many hours are you sleeping?" I asked him.

"Sometimes five, if I'm lucky," he said. "Today, for instance, I got in at 3 from work, the alarm went off at 7. I gulped two cups of black coffee and had to finish work on a twenty-page paper that was due at 12. Frankie wanted some loving, but to tell you the truth, I just couldn't get it up. And here I am."

"Well, for starters, an erection requires that many things be in place in order to get hard," I said. "One of the most important things you seem to be in short supply of is adequate sleep. When you are sleep-deprived, as you obviously are, and under the gun with other things that are due, it's difficult to focus on sex, let alone have the physiological state to make an erection happen. You just have too much distress in your life right now.

"My advice to you is to prioritize. Be more selfish with your time. Make sure that you get enough sleep, or as much as you can under these circumstances. You also need to speak with Frank. You have a tough schedule and he has to understand that. Good sex is only going to occur when you are rested and in the mood. If he really cares for you, he will be there for you when you are ready."

Zack finally smiled for the first time and stood up. "What you say makes a whole lot of sense. Thanks, Doctor," he said, and headed for the door. "You've taken a huge load off my mind."

SLEEP LESSONS

Lesson 1 Any factor that has a detrimental effect on your health will have a detrimental effect on your hardness.

Lesson 2 Sleep is as necessary as food and water for all people.

Lesson 3 Normal sleep patterns result in healthy nocturnal erections during the dream state.

WEEK FOUR   WEEK FIVE   WEEK SIX

SHORT CIRCUIT—PERSONAL BROWNOUTS

Do you find yourself tired, so much so that you are even too tired for sex? You are certainly not alone. Many men come to me complaining that they seem to be low on energy. Instead of getting any action in the bedroom, the sack has strictly been used for snoozing.

This week, I want you to examine the current state of your energy levels. Energy is simply the ability to do work—nothing more, nothing less. And when you possess it—whether it be the energy to get through the workday with plenty of pep left in your engine for an unexpected evening encounter, being able to throw together a dinner party for ten on the spur of the moment, or having the strength and stamina to shovel the snow from the driveway—you certainly know it. You are game to pursue just about anything. You are full of vitality. Your outlook is positive and no task seems daunting as you pursue all that life has to offer in a way that makes you feel fulfilled and happy.

GOING DOWN?

When energy levels are low, your posture slumps, along with just about everything else including your penis. You are just getting by—barely. Oftentimes, you become sick and depressed. I am sure you know many people who are totally lacking the desire and energy level to do anything. Some have just run out of steam—or so they have convinced themselves. Therefore, they just sit, day after day, waiting for something to happen instead of taking the initiative. It's this heightened inaction that becomes such a terrible habit that it takes a lot of effort to break.

There are many causes for lack of energy. The stress of everyday life is certainly high on the list, as are family matters, finances, and aging, with all its metabolic and physical changes. Nevertheless, after acknowledging the low energy ebb, a willingness to effect change and battle back from the energy deficit makes recovery possible and well worth the effort.

RENEWING YOUR ENERGY SOURCES

The most effective energy renewal plan I know of encompasses many factors. The more you adhere to the following suggestions, the better you can boost your energy. Here is my advice:

If you are always low on energy, find out why. Contact your physician. Men often feel this isn't worth a visit to the doctor, but it's an important marker of something being physically out of sync. Explain when it was that you first noticed the lack of energy. Did it come on the heels of the death of a loved one or after a bout with the flu? Be as clear as you can in detailing whether you feel sleepy or physically weak. Does your energy wax and wane throughout the day or week, or do you always feel sapped of energy?

Medications. They are, as previously mentioned, well-known energy drainers—especially antidepressants. If you are fatigued, or otherwise bereft of energy for two weeks or longer, it is a tip-off that something may be medically wrong. Some possibilities include depression, the onset of diabetes, or a heart or lung problem.

Keep stress under control. Stress is a stimulant, but if it is unrelenting, you are sapped of high energy, leaving you fatigued emotionally and physically. Studies continually report that stress is linked to 90 percent of all illnesses. While most people go out of their way to schedule and keep business meetings, they rarely schedule time or make appointments to take care of their emotional health. Physical touch has a positive impact on your emotional well-being and stress levels. A good stress buster can be something as simple as hugging your loved one. Find ways to reduce stress through relaxation techniques, regular exercise (did you walk today?), professional counseling, or a combination of the three.

Be active. Keep walking. You will feel more energetic when you are in good physical condition. A twenty-minute walk around the neighborhood each day is enough to get your motor revved.

Eat right. What you eat can play a big role in energy boosting and maintenance. Many people find that a breakfast and lunch high in protein rather than carbohydrates and fat is less apt to cause sluggishness. Avoid energy-sapping meals that are heavy in sugar. Although sugary foods trigger a quick energy infusion, your energy will soon desert you, leaving you feeling fatigued and listless.

> The physical reality of sex is about endurance, strength, balance, and agility.

Know yourself. Understand your individual energy cycle. For most people, energy normally peaks around noon; for others, it peaks later in the day. Once you know your own particular pattern, make changes in your schedule to accommodate it. For example, if you know that at 11 A.M. you are at your most energetic, schedule your most demanding mental and physical tasks for that time. Leave routine work for when your energy levels are naturally lower.

Do less. I get fatigued just listening to some of my patients as they describe a typical day. Some attempt to cram too many activities into their waking hours, resulting in a sure-fire energy drain before the sun sets. Who was it that said you had to go out to eat every night, join the twilight tennis league and the hiking club, and race off to Mexico for the weekend? Instead of spreading yourself so thin, scale back and choose one or two activities and pour all of your energy into them. You will get more enjoyment as well as a sense of fulfillment.

Pull the plug. Television is one of the greatest energy drainers. As you sit glued in front of the television for hours each week, inert except perhaps for the movement of hand-to-chips-to-mouth, your initiative to accomplish things quickly begins to seep into the fabric of the armchair.

Get out. A quick way to clear your mind and recharge your batteries is to drop everything and head outside. Better yet, go with your partner. Away

WEEK ONE   WEEK TWO   WEEK THREE

from the confines of your home or office, you have a chance to breathe in deep lungfuls of fresh air, feel the sun as it beats on your body, and just listen to the sounds of nature. Coming into contact with other people as you stroll is also a great energy booster.

Get a dog. Sure, there's going to be some hair to vacuum and slobber to clean from chairs and couches, but the companionship and the need to be walked several times a day will keep you moving and add variety to your life.

Laugh . . . a lot. One of the best energy boosters is laughter. A good laugh, whether it be to a series of one-liners or a zany movie, helps reduce stress and change your mood, and it leaves you feeling upbeat, the perfect scenario for an energy infusion.

PEYRONIE'S DISEASE—LIFE'S CURVEBALL

You're typically the first one to notice and it comes as a complete shock. Instead of projecting straight out when you have an erection, your penis now takes a decided curve to the side. In more advanced cases, the erection elicits pain and intercourse becomes problematic or impossible for you or your partner.

No, you don't have cancer of the penis, nor is it life threatening, as men once commonly thought. You most likely have what is known as Peyronie's (pa-ro-NEEZ) disease, an uncommon sexual dysfunction that results in a "bent" penis during erection. This disorder of the connective tissue within the penis causes the abnormal curvature during erection. While certainly not a new ailment, it's fairly rare—diagnosed in only 26 out of 100,000 men each year in the United States. In 1743, French surgeon Francois Gigot de Peyronie first described the penile curvature that bears his name. Not knowing the cause, doctors originally linked the unnatural bending to masturbation or some sexually transmitted disease.

What Peyronie's experts do know is that while the ailment is called a "disease," no precipitating cause has been found. Unlike many other diseases, Peyronie's cannot be transmitted from one person to another.

When it comes to treatment, there are many noninvasive medical treatments aimed at straightening the penis and relieving the pain that comes with an erection. Unfortunately, most are of limited value or simply do not work at all. Surgery and, in severe cases where erectile dysfunction is present, the implantation of a prosthetic device are reserved for those men who have extreme curvature, plaque formation, and pain.

Some men have either mild or partial erectile dysfunction predating Peyronie's disease; most men don't. Some researchers link Peyronie's to aging. The ailment primarily affects men between 40 and 60 years of age. Aging may diminish penile elasticity, increasing the chance of injury and the development of Peyronie's.

> **Chain of Command**
>
> A man's ejaculation consits of three separate bursts emanating from the Cowper's glands, the prostate, and finally the testicles.

When a man notices his erections are no longer straight, it's best that he consult with a physician. A urologist will induce a nonsexual erection pharmacologically in order to appraise penile rigidity and curvature. Management is then based on how bad the bend is, as well as erectile function. Penile-straightening surgery is recommended for the most severe cases.

Further trauma to the penis can be avoided by practicing "safe" sex. This means using copious amounts of lubricant during sex and avoiding all positions where the penis could possibly buckle during intercourse.

SENSUAL NUTRITION

I want you to adopt a more reasonable view of what to eat, taking care to consume a variety of foods—the best way to make sure you obtain a nutritionally balanced diet. In addition, I cannot stress enough that balancing your caloric intake with your caloric expenditure is the simple key to weight control. Whenever your caloric intake is greater than the amount of energy you use (you eat too much, exercise too little), any excess calories will be converted to body fat—and it makes little difference what nutritional package the extra calories happen to come in.

Here are two new recipes from Waldy
I want you to try this week

MENU ONE

ROASTED SHELLFISH STEW WITH TOMATOES AND GARLIC

Mediterranean Stuffed Zucchini with Cilantro-Yogurt Sauce
Roasted Shellfish Stew with Tomatoes and Garlic
Almond Ricotta Cake with Moscato-Roasted Apricots

MENU TWO

CRISP PENNE WITH RICOTTA, TOMATOES, AND HERBS

Roasted Clams with Garlic, Lemon, and Red Pepper
Crisp Penne with Ricotta, Tomatoes, and Herbs
Lemon Pudding Cakes with Persimmon
(See **Appendix II** for recipes)

SIX-WEEK PROGRAM

1. HARDNESS FACTOR

Rate your current level of hardness for Day Twenty-eight of the program. (Check off one box.)

○ Soft   ○ Soft/Hard   ○ Hard
○ Very Hard   ○ Like a Steel Beam

2. SEXUAL FITNESS

FROM WEEKS 1–3:

- Side Lunge Reach (15 repetitions)
- Angry Cat Stretch (3 times)
- Woodchopper Exercise (15 repetitions)

1. Bridge NEW

This stretches and strengthens the core muscles.

- Lie on your back, with your knees bent, feet flat on the floor and hip-width apart.
- Contract your abdominal muscles and buttocks and lift your hips off the floor toward the ceiling.
- Hold the raised bridge position for 3 seconds and then slowly lower your back down to the floor.
- Repeat 10 times.

FROM WEEKS 1–3:

- Classic Push-Ups (3 sets of 8 repetitions) or Modified Push-Ups (3 sets of 10 repetitions)
- Plank (4 sets, hold 45 seconds, rest 15 seconds)
- Cobra (10 repetitions)
- Squat (15 repetitions)

2. Squat Thrust NEW

This exercise promotes stability of the core, strengthens the chest and triceps, and improves the range of motion of your lower back and hips.

- Stand with your feet hip-width apart and your hands at your sides.
- Bend down and place your palms on the floor, shoulder-width apart, fingers pointed forward.
- Kick your feet back into a Classic Push-Up position and hold for 3 seconds.
- Contract your abdominal muscles, pull your knees back toward your hands, and then stand up.
- Repeat 3 times.

3. WALKING

Take 8,000 steps a day. Circle each day you achieved this goal:

Sunday   Monday   Tuesday   Wednesday
Thursday   Friday   Saturday

4. HARDNESS FACTOR SUPPLEMENTS

FROM WEEKS 1–3:
Take Pycnogenol (80 mg)/L-arginine (3 g) mixture or Pycnogenol Plus or Prelox Blue daily.

Horny Goat Weed (2 500-mg capsules)
Take 2 horny goat weed capsules daily.
Take 4 capsules one to two hours prior to a sexual encounter.

Take 2 Omega-3 Fatty Acid capsules.

1. Red Wine and Grape Seed Extract NEW
Take 200 mg of red wine extract and 100 mg of grape seed extract

5. SENSUAL NUTRITION

Shellfish

Shellfish are rich in a variety of B vitamins and vitamin E, both of which are great for heart and hardness. And don't forget that shellfish contain omega-3 fatty acids, which reduce the risk of heart disease.

Prepare two sensuous meals this week.

- Roasted Shellfish Stew with Tomatoes and Garlic
- Crisp Penne with Ricotta, Tomatoes, and Herbs

A MAN @ 45

Your lifestyle choices of the past twenty years are starting to show. If you took good care of your health, erections are hard and powerful.

More sexual stimulation is needed by many to achieve maximum hardness. Foreplay may become as important to you as it is for your partner.

The refractory period, the time between erections, is starting to increase.

If you have not taken good care of your health, prescription erection drugs may be a temporary recourse while trying to improve your hardness factor.

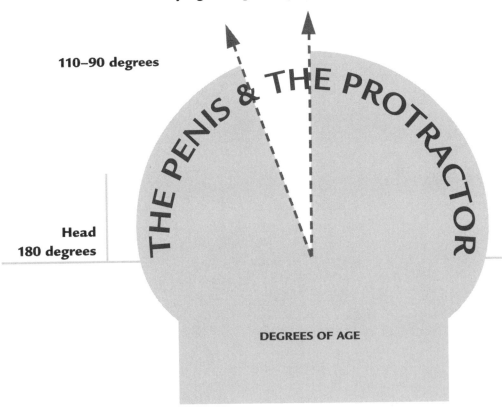

110–90 degrees

THE PENIS & THE PROTRACTOR

Head
180 degrees

Feet
0 degrees

DEGREES OF AGE

THE FOURTH WEEK—A HARD WEEK

Success can be measured in all the many little steps you have taken to bring about change in your life over the past twenty-eight days. Look how far you have come in your daily celebrations of good health and hardness.

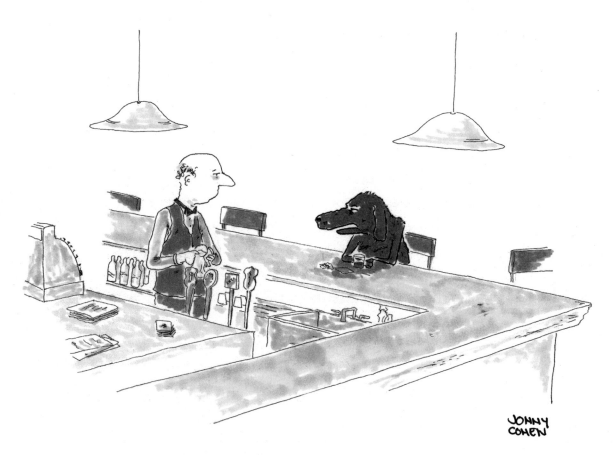

"THEN THE BITCH LEFT ME."

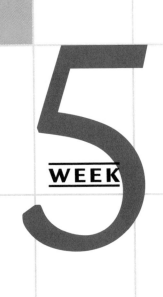

5
WEEK

Two more weeks to go. This week I want you to continue with all of the specific sexual fitness exercises you have been doing. You probably are recognizing that these "simple and easy" routines have become more challenging as they have increased. Don't be discouraged—you are a totally different person, harder with more stamina, and each new exercise or increased repetition brings you to another new place. Congratulations on laying the foundation for a "harder" lifestyle that you will be adhering to for the rest of your life.

8

YOU FEEL THE CHANGE AND SO DOES YOUR PENIS

Body image contributes greatly to your sex appeal. I am certain that your body image has changed for the better over the course of the past four weeks, and for some it has been a dramatic makeover. Your positive personal self-image will build self-confidence and enhance your hardness in the process. Your clothes should fit you differently, a new notch has been discovered on your belt, and you don't feel as tired. Any earlier hesitation about the strength of your erection should be a distant memory.

COMING TOGETHER

Evaluate your progress by how vital and energetic you now feel. Make a list of five goals you want to achieve this week. It's very satisfying to check each one off as you meet or exceed the goal. Success comes in small steps, not huge leaps. Come to the realization that these past four weeks have been a celebration of good health on the road to hardness and happiness.

The Fifth-Week Assignments

Sexual Fitness

▶ Increase walking to 9,000 steps a day this week. You are also going to work on strengthening thigh and hip muscles as well as augmenting flexibility through your hips with the Hip-Flexor Stretch and Single Leg Squat.

Hardness Factor Supplements

▶ Your goal this week is to begin raising your level of good cholesterol, your HDL. Start by taking 2 400-mg capsules of non-flush niacin, a supplement that increases HDL more than any other.

Sensual Nutrition

▶ Learn how to safely lose weight and keep it off forever. It starts by understanding the basics of metabolism and learning not to fear calories.

Erection Rx

▶ Contrary to popular belief, it is not always the woman who is infertile. Getting a woman pregnant depends on maximum hardness and plenty of healthy sperm. Learn what you can do to maximize your sperm production this week.

When It's Harder to Get Hard, Tell Your Doctor

FRANK, age 47— I'm not having an affair, I'm having a heart attack

Nicole was in for a flu shot, but she seemed distracted. I sensed there was something she wanted to discuss. At 38, this vibrant television producer was a head turner, with her mass of red curls that hung to her shoulders and a toned body made fit by daily loops in Central Park and Bikram yoga sessions. "One more thing, if you have a moment," she said tentatively, gathering her things to leave. "It's about Frank, actually. Something is not right with him and it has me upset. He went to his doctor and he gave him a prescription for Cialis. Frank's doctor told him it was natural at his age, just part of life and aging."

I urged Nicole to sit back down. I knew her husband, Frank, as a man in the glare of the national spotlight. A successful entrepreneur, with several ventures that merited extensive articles in the financial press over the past few years, 47-year-old Frank didn't strike me as a man to upset his mild-mannered wife. Married for three years, theirs was a second marriage for both. "Tell me about your concerns," I said.

"This is all so intimate," she said, exhaling softly. "Okay. At first, I thought Frank was having an affair. We haven't had sex for more than half a year because Frank is embarrassed that his erection isn't as hard as it was—sometimes it just disappears. I don't want to make him feel bad so I sort of ignore it." Nicole blushed after this revelation. "When the Cialis didn't seem to make much of a difference it really scared me. Frank didn't say much at all. Ever since then, he hasn't shown any interest sexually. And it's not just the sex part that I miss. It's hard to even get him to cuddle with me at night. It's as if a part of him just died. And this from a man who couldn't keep his hands off me. No more, though. Frank says nothing is wrong, but Doctor, I know there is. Do you think he is seeing someone else or maybe he's gay?"

A bell goes off whenever I hear that there has been a change in a man's typical sexual patterns, whether it be his libido or monthly rate of sexual intercourse. The change in a man's sexual appetite or interest in intercourse can be troubling for a partner. "When a man who has always been ready and able to perform is suddenly not able to or is just not interested, other body parts may hold the answer," I told Nicole. "I doubt that his sexual orientation has changed or that there is another woman. If you can get him to come to see me, I will find the underlying cause of this. That's a promise."

As an internist, I'm witness to the dangers men face on a daily basis when they deny they have a health issue. According to the National Center for Health Statistics, women make 471 million office visits a year compared to 316 million visits logged by men. That's 3.5 visits per year for women and 2.4 for men. The bottom line is that many men are often hurting—mentally and physically—yet they don't seek help. They don't give themselves permission to explore their medical concerns.

Men like Frank are in denial—or simply don't know better—when they ignore the connection between hardness failures and their health. I felt the same could be said for the doctor who had prescribed Cialis for Frank. In defense of this physician, however, your typical doctor will generally not suspect that a man approaching 50 might have erectile dysfunction related to heart disease, and instead he will write off his hardness complaints to either a temporary stress-related incident or the beginning of andropause.

This is especially true when the patient is not forthcoming with pertinent information. For example, Frank had neglected to mention that he was often short of breath walking up the flight of stairs in his duplex apartment.

Unfortunately, a golden opportunity is missed because many times ED = ED; that is, erectile dysfunction equals *endothelial* dysfunction. In laymen's terms: Erectile dysfunction is often a sign of problems with the endothelium, the lining of the blood vessels. The vessels may be inflamed due to a large plaque buildup and ready to send a lethal clot into an artery of the heart. Though sexual medicine has been one of the most significant impacts in men's health there is also a danger of treating a symptom and not the disease.

Frank, who is six feet two and weighs 218 pounds, was in to see me the next day. He told me that he usually ended a challenging day at the office at 9 p.m., and then headed straight to the company gym to lift weights and use the elliptical trainer before going home.

He had been following this routine for almost two years. Thanks in part to a dramatic shift in his eating habits under Nicole's guidance, he had also trimmed away twenty-five pounds of flab. Unfortunately, most of these well-intentioned lifestyle changes had fallen to the wayside over the past year due to a business slump that kept him at his desk. The weight was coming back on, as were the martinis that he drank to calm his nerves.

"And besides, I just felt too tired to exercise like I used to," he told me. "I would often get fatigued and quickly out of breath, but I chalked it up to the late hours needed to get one of my companies back on track," Frank said. "I never told Nicole any of this. I don't want to worry her."

Frank finally told me he could get an erection but it wasn't firm, even with the help of a prescription drug. This was something he just attributed to overwork and incredible levels of stress in his life. His last really hard erection, he recalled, was almost eight months ago.

> 66 Frank finally told me he could get an erection but it wasn't firm, even with the help of a prescription drug.

Granted, all of that was certainly possible, I told Frank. And even though Frank looked like he was fairly healthy I suspected something else: heart disease.

With an inability to get an erection and now with an acknowledgment that over the past months he felt a growing tightness in his chest and shortness of breath, I thought that Frank was actually at high risk of a heart attack. I picked up the phone and called a cardiologist to make an appointment for Frank the next day.

Frank's symptoms, including the failure of hardness, were part of a cry for help from arteries in his heart and elsewhere that weren't able to get enough oxygenated blood through his plaque-clogged vessels. The condition worsened when Frank tried to exercise, which brought on the breathlessness and chest pain. Unfortunately, the years before Nicole's intervention of fat-laden foods, late night business dinners, post-dinner cigars, and little or no exercise trumped his recent attempts at a health makeover,

WEEK FOUR   *WEEK FIVE*   WEEK SIX

especially with the recent backsliding. Adding to the negative column was heart disease in his family. His father and older brother both died from heart attacks before the age of 60.

It turned out that Frank had a cholesterol level of 220, which was high but not uncommon. Moreover, his extremely low HDL level of 19 put him in the "at risk" category for heart disease. The exercise stress test he then took on the treadmill was "strongly positive" for heart blockage. Several days later Frank had an angiogram. In this procedure, a catheter was threaded from his groin up into his heart, affording the cardiac specialist a chance to look closely at his arteries. Three major arteries and a small tributary were found to be 85 percent blocked.

CABG (pronounced "cabbage"), or coronary artery bypass graft surgery, was performed the following week to redirect blood flow around Frank's clogged arteries.

Frank had dodged a big bullet. With youth and relative good health in his favor, he came through the surgery just fine. Eight weeks later and 20 pounds lighter, he was back to see me at my office. He had resumed his daily exercise and was now on a low-salt, low-fat diet.

I told Frank that even though his heart had been repaired, allowing for increased cardiac output and more blood flow to his penis, we still had to deal with the underlying atherosclerosis that was present in his penile blood vessels and the rest of his body.

"Dr. Lamm, I don't know if it was a mental or a physical reaction, but a few days after my surgery I woke up with an erection, a hard erection. Sex is back in my life, which is great," Frank said. "Mine really is a story that comes with a 'happy ending,' like the one I had last night," he said. His smile was all that was needed to understand his meaning.

HEART-BREAKING LESSONS

Lesson 1   Men in their 40s can have severe erectile problems.

Lesson 2   Men in their 40s can have severe coronary artery disease (CAD). CAD can be "silent," with the first manifestation being sudden death for about 750,000 Americans. The "lucky" ones will have overt symptoms of shortness of breath and/or chest pain and can be helped by their doctors.

Lesson 3   Failure to respond to one prescription erection medication is not a reason to switch to another drug. Rather, it is a reason to be evaluated by your doctor as soon as possible for serious underlying medical problems.

Lesson 4   Be honest with your physician when describing hardness problems. By understanding all of your complaints and symptoms, your doctor will be able to make a more accurate diagnosis, possibly saving your life in the process.

Lesson 5   Just because your heart has been revitalized through surgical intervention with coronary artery bypass surgery or an angioplasty and stenting, the rest of your blood vessels are still at risk. Pay attention to what you eat and how much you exercise. If your doctor prescribes statin medication, be sure to take it daily.

HEART DISEASE CHECKLIST

Heart attacks can develop without warning. However, there are often tell-tale warning signs that may appear years in advance. If you have any of the following warning signs of underlying heart disease, consult your doctor. Ignoring warning signs of heart disease can be fatal. Being aware of the following common symptoms of heart disease and initiating effective treatment will help prevent more serious problems from developing.

1. Decreased hardness As plaque builds up in the arteries and vessels, optimal blood flow to the penis is reduced, resulting in a softer erection. Speak to your doctor at the first signs of hardness diminution.

2. High blood pressure and high blood cholesterol Elevated blood pressure and elevated blood cholesterol are both warning signs of possible underlying heart problems. Both conditions can be treated by your doctor with medication and lifestyle modification.

3. Angina Angina, or chest pain, is a temporary pain, pressure, or tightness in your chest that occurs when your heart muscles are being deprived of oxygenated blood. The pain or discomfort may travel to your throat or jaw, lower back, or to your left shoulder or arm.

    Stable angina is chest pain that occurs when you exercise and disappears at rest.

    Unstable angina occurs unexpectedly at rest. If you experience unstable angina, contact your doctor immediately. **A heart attack may be imminent.**

4. Shortness of breath Shortness of breath is the most common symptom of heart disease. Heart failure doesn't mean your heart has stopped working, but rather that your heart is struggling to pump enough blood for your body. When this occurs, there is fluid buildup in the lungs, which makes breathing difficult.

5. Swollen legs and feet Swelling in the legs, ankles, and feet is due to the collection of fluid in the tissues. This is another symptom of heart failure.

6. Pain in the legs when walking Pain in the calf muscles when you walk is called claudication. This is a symptom of narrowed blood vessels in the leg, and is often a sign that there are also blockages of arteries in the heart.

NOTE: If you have one or more of these heart disease symptoms, contact your doctor immediately.

BOOSTING HDL BOOSTS HARDNESS

Total cholesterol blood levels, which are based on a combination of LDL and HDL readings, should be less than 200 mg/dL. However, researchers now believe that upward of 25 million Americans with healthy cholesterol scores are actually at risk for heart problems because their HDL levels are too low.

It is important that men get their HDL levels to the highest level possible. With every 1-unit increase in HDL, heart disease risk drops by as much as 3 percent. As I explained to Jim, a 31-year-old patient who needed to raise his HDL from a subpar 39 by getting his HDL up to 45, he would decrease his chance of heart disease by more than 15 percent.

Raising HDL pays huge dividends. When you get your HDL up, your hardness potential increases with it. I always advise any man concerned with achieving and maintaining optimal erectile functioning to begin exploring all of the steps that can help get his number up. The following eight lifestyle measures can make a big difference:

1. Exercise.

Exercising is the single most effective way of raising HDL levels, and it will reduce your overall risks of erectile problems and heart disease.

A study published recently in *Circulation* reported that men with heart conditions who pedaled a stationary bike for 20 minutes a day had significantly higher levels of HDL after one year than another group of men with heart conditions who did no exercise at all. In fact, the HDL levels of the nonexercisers actually plummeted.

The 10,000-step daily walking program you are on and the daily sexual fitness exercises that you are performing are certainly going to help boost your HDLs.

2. Lose weight.

If you are overweight, slimming down through a combination of exercising and eating a healthier, well-balanced diet is essential. Obesity is doubly

WEEK FOUR   *WEEK FIVE*   WEEK SIX

dangerous for the heart and penis because it promotes higher levels of "bad" cholesterol and lower levels of HDL cholesterol.

3. Quit smoking.

If that nasty smoker's breath does not kill your chances of success in the bedroom, the damage that smoking does to your heart and lungs is guaranteed to do the job eventually. Smoking lowers HDL levels by an average of 4 mg/dL, and it also increases LDL levels. Stop smoking now and watch your HDL start to rise.

4. Have a drink.

Alcohol, taken moderately, can significantly raise your HDL levels. Just remember that anything more than one or two drinks a day will do more harm than good. Taking your red wine extract daily can certainly help here as well. I happen to prefer red wine extract to the alcohol—it's easier to control the dosage and it's also noncaloric.

5. Reduce saturated fats.

The saturated fats found in meat, dairy products, and coconut oil, as well as the trans-fatty acids used in many prepared foods to increase shelf life, all lower HDL levels while raising your "bad" cholesterol count.

Whenever possible, substitute with the polyunsaturated fats found in sunflower and safflower oil or, better still, the monounsaturated fats found in olive oil and canola oil. Monounsaturated fats can actually boost HDL levels, so the switch will be well worth any inconvenience.

6. Add fiber to your diet.

Two servings a day of the soluble fiber found in oats, fruits, and vegetables will not only keep you regular, they will improve your cholesterol profile. Just eating oatmeal at breakfast can make a dramatic improvement in your cholesterol and it also may explain why that guy is always smiling on the box.

7. Load up on antioxidants.

Cholesterol molecules are highly vulnerable to oxidation, and this damaging process can interfere with HDL cholesterol's ability to transport "bad" cholesterol back to the liver for destruction. Pycnogenol, red wine and grape seed extracts, blueberries, strawberries, and dark green vegetables all play valuable roles. Vitamin C and E supplements will also help protect and maintain your HDL level. See Week Six for the complete C and E supplement program.

8. Supplement with niacin.

This supplement will significantly boost HDL.

> 66 When you get your HDL up, your hardness potential also goes up.

NIACIN WORKS VERY HARD

Taking as little as twenty-five cents' worth of niacin, which is sometimes called vitamin B$_3$, per day can be an extremely potent weapon in the battle to boost HDL levels.

In the 1950s, niacin was found to improve cholesterol levels when taken in large doses, making it the oldest known medication we have for treating cholesterol problems. Recent studies have shown that niacin actually promotes regression of hardened arteries, rejuvenating the blood vessels and increasing the amount of blood that is pumped into the penile arteries—blood needed to significantly increase your hardness.

Niacin occurs naturally in fruits, vegetables, meats, and whole grains, but in order to ingest enough of it to have a positive effect on the heart and penis, supplements need to be added to your diet. Doses of between 400 milligrams and 1,000 milligrams a day can boost HDL levels significantly, lowering "bad" cholesterol levels in the bargain. Taking even higher doses of 2 grams or more, only under the supervision of your physician, will produce dramatic boosts in HDL levels.

WEEK FOUR   *WEEK FIVE*   WEEK SIX

OH, QUIT BLUSHING—REDUCING SIDE EFFECTS

Some of my patients have experienced an uncomfortable heat, facial flushing, and/or itching on the upper body while taking niacin supplements in the 1,000 milligram (1 gram) range. In rare instances, gastrointestinal upset and lightheadedness can also occur, as well as liver function abnormalities or a temporary rise in blood sugar. All of these side effects generally lessen over time, however, as the body acclimates to the presence of high levels of niacin in the bloodstream.

Some patients find that taking one "baby" aspirin tablet (81 milligrams) about thirty minutes before taking the supplements reduces any unwanted side effects, as does taking them with a meal. Additionally, taking niacin right before going to bed may be helpful, as any side effects that occur will pass unnoticed during the sleep cycle.

Several companies now offer no-flush niacin supplements. By delivering a steady stream of niacin over the course of several hours rather than having the entire dose dumped into the bloodstream at once, many of the potential side effects are minimized, if not eliminated altogether. Take care not to crush, break, or chew any brand of no-flush extended-release niacin tablets, as this will undermine their ability to slowly release the vitamin into your bloodstream.

THE HARDNESS FACTOR NIACIN PROGRAM

Because the dietary supplement **niacin is not regulated** by the FDA, the **amount** of niacin in the products **varies widely** from none at all to much more than labeled. **High doses** of niacin can be **harmful** and require a doctor's supervision.

Start the niacin program after you have had a **blood test** and know what your **HDL level** is. Ideally, I like to see men have HDL levels in the **60 mg/dL range** because that is where most of the heart protection kicks in.

If you have an HDL level that is already in a **good range (40 mg/dL or slightly higher,** as determined by your blood test), take **1 400-mg** no-flush niacin capsule **daily.**

If your doctor has told you that your HDL levels are **low** and **should be raised,** niacin will help you achieve that goal. Doses of **1–2 grams** of niacin a day can **raise HDL** by as much as **35 percent** and **lower triglycerides** by up to **50 percent.** Speak to your doctor about taking these very high doses of niacin so you can achieve the maximum heart and penis protection.

The niacin that I have recommended to my patients is Res-Q HDL +, manufactured by N3 Oceanic, the same company that manufactures the omega-3 capsules I discussed in Week Three. The prescription product Niaspan is also an excellent product.

Check the Hardness Factor Shopping List (page 327) for recommended niacin supplements.

SENSUAL NUTRITION

I am not a fan of diets. I want you to get the word *diet* out of your lexicon and replace it with "healthful eating." Diets are hard to maintain because they usually require you to give up your favorite foods. At some point—a few weeks for some, only a few days for others—most people simply give up and go back to their old eating habits. That is, until another best-selling diet book comes along with its hyped-up claims of easy weight loss and new eating regimens.

The battle to lose excess inches and pounds of unwanted body fat is a problem common to the estimated 10 million Americans on some form of weight reduction program. Unfortunately, jumping diets from Atkins to South Beach to the Hamptons in hopes of instant results is endemic among most long-term dieters. This is why the national success rate for any diet is ultimately an abysmally low 8 percent.

Cut back slightly on your eating and expend an additional 200 calories each day (minimum) in some form of physical activity—a brisk forty-minute walk, a session on your stairclimber, some swimming—and you will be making a substantial effort in reducing your excess weight. Since you are now in Week Five of the program, you have more than likely noticed that already. As you continue with your walking over a period of months, you will not only feel better, but look better as well. Don't be surprised if someone starts calling you "sexy" soon.

SKIP THE NUMBERS GAME

Weighing yourself every day or two to check your results is definitely counterproductive for a couple of reasons: Weight fluctuates daily due to fluid retention. One day you might register a loss of two pounds and the next be up three—and ready to throw in the towel on your weight-reduction regime.

Second, and more important if you are (as you should be) exercising daily and cutting back on your caloric intake, you might start to look and feel slimmer without actually registering any weight loss. This is because muscle cells weigh more than fat cells. Therefore, while you're converting the unwanted fat into leaner muscle, the gauge on the bathroom scale might not be dropping. Don't be discouraged. Weigh yourself less frequently, and with time you'll see the pounds coming off.

EATING FOR ENJOYMENT AND HEALTH

Wholesome meals are too often neglected in the rush and stresses of everyday life. While your walking program may be squeezed into an already hectic schedule, proper nutrition often is squeezed out. That's a big mistake. If there's one thing an active person should not neglect, it's keeping the body well fueled with nutritious food throughout the day.

Don't skip breakfast or lunch or else you're likely to end up with a ravenous appetite in the evening and may be tempted to eat everything in sight, making all the wrong food choices in the process. When you're very hungry, you don't care about choices—you're just looking for something quick and easy. If you're not prepared, this could end up being a big bag of chips or a pint of chocolate ice cream. This is much less likely to happen if you make eating a good breakfast and lunch a priority.

> Failure to achieve a daily erection may be cause for alarm.

By eating these two meals, you provide your body with the calories it needs to work or walk. Go without them and you'll end up standing in front of your refrigerator at night grabbing anything you can. You may regret it a half-hour after binging on cookies or candy—but then it's too late.

BREAKFAST, EVERYONE?

Make a commitment to eating a solid breakfast every morning. Many people with tight schedules think they don't have time to eat breakfast, but all it takes is a little planning. If you've put in your morning walk before heading off to work, or if you've gotten out of bed at the last possible minute before racing out the door, make plans to eat on the run. Breakfast doesn't have to be an elaborate, sit-down affair. It can be as simple as a bran muffin, yogurt, and a banana. The important thing is that you take in some food at this time.

If you prefer not to walk on an empty stomach, grab a light snack—a piece of toast, some crackers, or a glass of juice—before your walk, then have a more complete breakfast later.

LUNCH WITH A PUNCH

Lunch for the harried worker can also be as nutritious and simple to prepare as breakfast. Setting aside fifteen or thirty minutes to eat lunch is not a waste of time. Eating helps you sharpen your mental sword and is an investment in your afternoon performance, both physical and mental. Soup, a tuna sandwich, and some fruit are fine. If you want to eat at your desk, bring in a box of stoned wheat crackers, some peanut butter, and a piece of fruit, and you'll have all that you need for a heart-healthy meal.

DINNER—IT'S ALL IN THE TIMING

For many people, dinner follows closely on the heels of work and workouts. If you've eaten carefully during the day, this meal doesn't have to be packed with calories or require tremendous preparation.

If you find that your weekday schedule is hectic and you arrive home late, it's best to set aside a few hours on the weekend for snack and meal preparation. By washing, cleaning, and slicing fruit and vegetables ahead of time, there will always be something readily available throughout the week when you come home.

If your favorite fruit is out of season, try unsweetened frozen fruit or dried fruit. Alternatively, to be adventurous, try some different fruits that are in season. If you want to try canned fruit, make sure it's packed in its own natural juices. If it has a heavy sugar-based syrup, drain it off to save on empty sugar calories.

> *Here are two sensuous dinner recipes*
> *I want you to try this week*

《⦿MENU ONE

PEPPERED TUNA WITH RED WINE AND SHALLOTS

Seared Polenta Squares with Spicy Broccoli Rabe
Peppered Tuna with Red Wine and Shallots
Raspberry Cake

《⦿MENU TWO

VENISON CHOPS WITH SPICY CURRANT AND RED WINE SAUCE

Roasted Butternut Squash and Pear Soup
Venison Chops with Spicy Currant and Red Wine Sauce
Apple Crisps
(See **Appendix II** for recipes)

UNDERSTANDING YOUR BMR

The critical player in the weight game is called basal metabolic rate. It's also sometimes called resting metabolic rate, or RMR. What you need to know is that "basal" means at baseline, relaxed, or resting. "Metabolism" refers to the chemical processes in your body that provide energy for the maintenance of life.

"Basal metabolism" basically means how fast your body uses calories to maintain the function of vital organs such as your brain, heart, liver, lungs, and kidneys. Basal metabolism, which I measure in my office with special equipment as the number of calories-per-minute-per-kilogram of body weight utilized, is lowest upon awaking and highest during vigorous activities. Therefore, the more you exercise, the more calories you burn, the more weight you lose.

Great and Not-So-Great Apes

The mighty gorilla has a two-inch penis, while the privates of the chimpanzee measure three inches. Of all the primates, man has the largest penis. Out in the ocean, it is a different matter altogether. The blue whale has the largest penis in the animal kingdom: 11 feet.

In lieu of medical access to special equipment, here is an unscientific way of determining your current basal metabolism: Simply multiply your current weight by 10. For example, if you weigh 200 pounds, your BMR is 2,000.

Basal metabolic rate accounts for 70 percent of your daily calories, which proves that almost everyone uses more energy just living than they ever do while exercising. But here is an interesting point: One pound of fat burns about 2 calories per day. One pound of muscle burns as many as 50 calories per day. You readily boost your BMR when you pack on the muscle and lose the fat. This keeps your metabolic fires stoked to the maximum.

Between the ages of 20 and 40, a physically inactive man can easily gain seven or more pounds of fat, lose seven pounds of muscle, and develop a 7 percent slower metabolic rate, even though his weight stays the same. Does the bathroom scale lie? Not exactly. But it certainly does not tell the whole story.

BMR Facts You Need to Know

▶ Basal metabolism can vary considerably from one person to another. In general, large people tend to burn more calories than smaller people do, and people with large muscles burn calories faster than people of equal weight, but with a larger proportion of body fat.

▶ Many people believe that metabolism drops as you age, making you more susceptible to weight gain. Yes, it's true that basal metabolic rate tends to decrease starting at about age 30, but this decline is almost entirely due to a drop in muscle mass directly related to physical inactivity.

▶ Your metabolism does not have to drop, and you do not need to gain body fat. The best way to increase your metabolic rate is to decrease the amount of fat you are carrying and replace it with muscle. This calls for a combination of regular exercise—

your daily 10,000 steps—and sensible eating. Maintain lean body mass and you should have very few changes in your metabolism—at least until you reach your 70s, 80s, or beyond.

DON'T JUDGE A BOOK BY ITS COVER

When you want to have a baby, getting hard is half of the equation. Making sure you are fertile is the second part. In 50 percent of cases where couples are having difficulty conceiving a baby, the male partner is a major factor.

Houston, Do We Have a Problem?

ROB, age 30—Swimming upstream

I could see that Rob was clearly distraught. For almost six months, the 30-year-old account executive and his 28-year-old wife, Cheryl, had been trying to get pregnant. Cheryl had checked out okay with her gynecologist. After a thorough examination, her doctor said if there was a problem conceiving, the infertility issue was probably with Rob, not with Cheryl.

Rob, who exercised regularly and was conscientious about his diet, found it difficult to believe that he might be the cause of their failure to conceive. Although women have shouldered the blame for infertility for centuries, we now know that at least a significant percentage of the problems are directly related to the male. Rob brightened when I told him that if he was actually found to be infertile, the problem might easily be reversed, either with lifestyle modifications, medication, or a special minimally invasive surgical procedure. The urologist I was sending him to for a fertility workup would first look for evidence of excess heat to the testicles or any blockage in the prostate gland.

TO BE CONTINUED ▶

DOWNWARD MOTILITY

Sperm, the male reproductive cell, takes seventy-two days to grow in the testicles, which are naturally kept at a temperature 3 to 5 degrees below the normal body temperature of 98.6. More than 60 to 80 million sperm are produced with each ejaculation, with the head of each sperm containing the important genetic information, and the tail helping it move from vagina to uterus.

You Say Mobile, I Say Motile

Sperm motility is the percentage of all moving sperm in a semen sample. At least 50 percent or more should be moving rapidly.

Sperm count is indicative of the overall health of a man. Unfortunately, men do a lot of bad things to harm their sperm production without even realizing it. For instance, tight underwear increases temperature to less-than-optimal levels for sperm production. Sperm die off when exposed to high heat, so if you luxuriate in a hot tub, the heated water will damage sperm and reduce sperm levels for the next ninety days. Smoke cigarettes, drink excessively, use recreational drugs or anabolic steroids, and sperm can become misshapen, making fathering a child much more difficult.

Rob's urologist performed a semen analysis to check the number of sperm and also his sperm morphology, which would determine specifically how the heads were shaped and the action of the tails. Rob's sperm count was 25 million, which was low, and his sperm quality was not the best. Many of the sperm tails appeared bent, which made it difficult for them to move properly.

The doctor then examined his scrotum to see if he had a varicocele, a cluster of enlarged veins in the scrotum that can cause blood to pool and significantly raise the temperature in the testicles. These veins, which are found in approximately 40 percent of infertile males, are similar to varicose veins in the legs. Varicoceles are the most common cause of male infertility. Men with varicoceles can certainly be fertile but the heat they generate can damage sperm production, shape, and ability to move.

► *THE STORY CONTINUES*

ROB, age 30—Still swimming

Rob's urologist eventually discovered a varicocele and recommended minimally invasive surgery. While the procedure could not totally guarantee increased fertility, the doctor explained that approximately half of all repairs result in an eventual pregnancy.

In addition to varicoceles, a childhood illness such as mumps can negatively influence sperm production and cause fertility problems. Certain prescription medications used to treat high blood pressure can also cause problems, but sperm usually recover when the drugs are discontinued or switched. Infections, which can easily be treated by antibiotics, cause 20 percent of male fertility problems. In addition, blockages in the prostate can cause swelling and prevent sperm from exiting properly, a problem that can often be treated with medication.

Just because a man has been told that he is infertile does not mean that he will not be able to become a father. Gather all the information that you can and seek out a male fertility specialist. Rob opted for the varicocele procedure on an outpatient basis, which was covered by his insurance, and within months his sperm looked normal. Eight months later Cheryl got pregnant.

SWIMMING LESSONS	
Lesson 1	Sperm production can be affected by factors that may be independent of sexual drive and performance.
Lesson 2	Testicular trauma resulting from an injury can cause an immune response in the testes that can damage sperm. Your testicles need to be treated with TLC.

SIX-WEEK PROGRAM

1. HARDNESS FACTOR

Rate your current level of hardness for Day Thirty-five of the program. (Check off one box.)

○ Soft   ○ Soft/Hard   ○ Hard
○ Very Hard   ○ Like a Steel Beam

2. SEXUAL FITNESS

FROM WEEKS 1–4:

- Side Lunge Reach (**15 repetitions**)
- Angry Cat Stretch (**3 times**)
- Woodchopper Stretch (**20 repetitions**)
- Bridge (**15 repetitions**)

1. Hip-Flexor Stretch NEW

Most people have tight hip-flexors, so this will enhance flexibility, help prevent back discomfort, test balance, and improve core stability.

- Stand erect, feet together, hands at your sides.
- Take a step forward with your right foot, bending your right knee until your left knee is touching the floor.
- Contract your abdominal muscles and lean forward to gently stretch the front of the left hip flexor.
- Hold the stretch for 15 seconds.
- Repeat with the opposite leg.

FROM WEEKS 1–4:

- Classic Push-Ups (**3 sets of 10 repetitions**)*
- Plank (**5 sets, hold 60 seconds, rest 15 seconds**)
- Cobra (**10 repetitions**)
- Squat (**20 repetitions**)
- Squat Thrust (**5 repetitions**)

* If you've been doing Modified Push-Ups, it's time to graduate to the Classic Push-Up. Start with Week 1 sets and repetitions.

2. Single-Leg Squat NEW

An excellent exercise to improve balance, core integrity, quadricep and buttock strength, and ankle, knee, and hip coordination.

- Stand next to a chair or wall for balance when performing this exercise for the first time.
- Stand on your right leg with the foot pointing straight ahead and your left knee slightly bent, foot off the floor.
- Keep your weight distributed evenly over your right foot.
- Keep your upper body erect with your head facing forward.
- Bend from your right hip, knee, and ankle and touch your right shin with both hands while keeping your abdominals drawn into the spine.
- Return to the starting position.
- **Repeat 5 times with each leg.**

WEEK Five

3. WALKING

Take 9,000 steps a day. Circle each day you achieved this goal:

Sunday Monday Tuesday Wednesday
Thursday Friday Saturday

4. HARDNESS FACTOR SUPPLEMENTS

FROM WEEKS 1–4:
Pycnogenol (80 mg)/L-arginine (3 g) mixture or Pycnogenol Plus or Prelox Blue daily.

2 horny goat weed capsules daily.

2 Omega-3 fatty acid capsules daily.

Red wine (200 mg) and grape seed extract (100mg) daily.

1. Niacin
Take 2 400-mg no-flush niacin pills if your HDL level is in a good range. Speak to your doctor about higher doses if HDL levels are low.

5. SENSUAL NUTRITION

Fresh tuna, which looks almost like beef when it is raw, is naturally high in protein (good for muscle-building) and low in fat. Recent research has shown that omega-3 fatty acids, found in abundance in fatty fish like tuna, can help lower the risk of heart disease and stroke.

Venison (deer meat) may not be on your menu many times during the year, but this meat is high in protein and minerals and lower in fat and cholesterol than beef and other meats, and it is certainly a delicious centerpiece to a sensuous dining experience.

Prepare two sensuous meals this week.
- Peppered Tuna with Red Wine and Shallots
- Venison Chops with Spicy Currant and Red Wine Sauce

A MAN @ 55

A healthy lifestyle has preserved and enhanced your hardness. You are still performing at optimal levels.

The refractory period is increasing.

Hardness is negatively affected for those who have neglected their health over the years; restoration with prescription medication is inevitable for many.

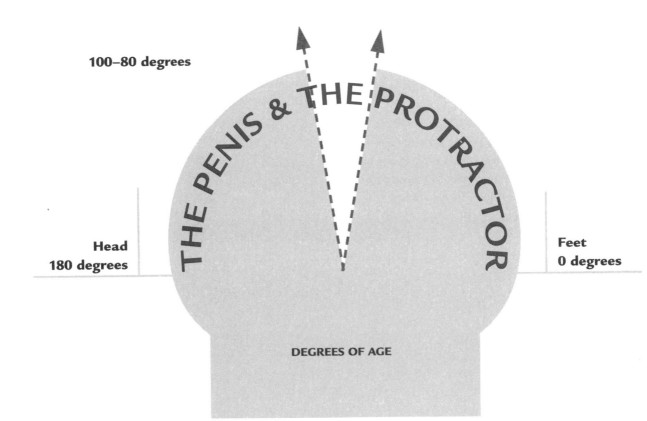

100–80 degrees

THE PENIS & THE PROTRACTOR

Head
180 degrees

Feet
0 degrees

DEGREES OF AGE

THE FIFTH WEEK—HARD IS GOOD

There is nothing like a home-cooked meal to set the table for romance. You have already been presented with almost one dozen new recipes over the past five weeks from master chef Waldy Malouf, and I hope you have had the chance to reestablish a new relationship with food during the course of the program.

I am not here to tell you what to eat but rather to encourage you to make use of these recipes as a surefire way to add enjoyment to your eating and maintain your hardness and good health.

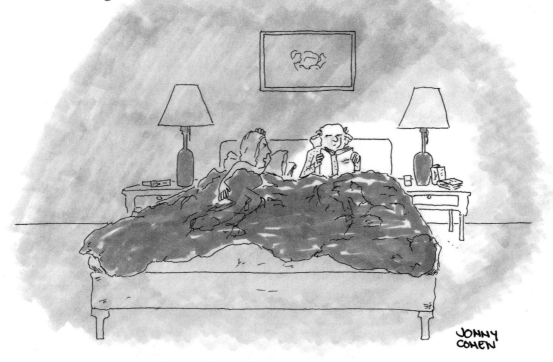

"I'M THE FEMININE SIDE YOU NEED TO GET IN TOUCH WITH."

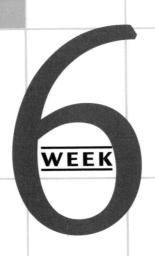

WEEK

You did it. This is the final week of the program. You have certainly come a long way in such a relatively short period. Look back at all of the positive changes you have made so far in the way that you live your life, in the ways you have enhanced your health and hardness, and in the ways that have added to the intimacy with your partner.

Review what you have particularly liked about the program. Either follow the program as I have laid it out for you, or else add your own modifications that you will be able to follow in the upcoming weeks, months, and years.

9

HARDNESS—A WAY OF LIFE

There are just a few more items to add to the program this week. By this time, you have come to appreciate the changes brought by the exercises, the supplements, and the nutritional recommendations. You have found ways to make them a part of your life. Your goal is hardness and health and following the program will help keep you on that solid path.

BETTER SEX, BETTER HEALTH, BETTER LIFE

Be honest. After five weeks, I am sure you have come to the realization that this is a program that doesn't just stop at the end of this week. Keep up all the good measures you have added to your life this week. Make the decision now to continue with the program. You have already made major strides in enhancing health and hardness. There is no reason to ever stop. Why would you want to?

The Final-Week Assignments

Sexual Fitness

▶ You finally reach your **10,000**-step landmark this week. For those who have been walking this far already, congratulations. Adding the additional **1,000** steps should be no problem for everyone else because I am sure you have already found many creative ways of incorporating movement into your day. For exercises, I have added a good neck stretch guaranteed to remove the kinks some of you may develop after performing oral sex, and two more stretches for your abdominals, back, chest, and shoulders.

Hardness Factor Supplements

▶ Pycnogenol (80 mg)/L-arginine (3 g) mixture or Pycnogenol Plus or Prelox Blue

▶ 2 horny goat weed capsules

▶ 2 Omega-3 fatty acid capsules

▶ Red wine (200 mg) and grape seed extract (100 mg)

▶ 2 400-mg no-flush niacin pills if your HDL level is in a good range; speak to your doctor about higher doses if HDL levels are low

Vitamins C and E

Take 500 mg of vitamin C and 200–400 IU of vitamin E.

Sensual Nutrition

The nutritional recommendations I have offered are not that difficult to incorporate into your busy life. Let's briefly review these suggestions simply as a handy reminder of the foods that will enhance hardness.

▶ In Week One, you learned how to steer away from a variety of foods that negatively impact heart health and hardness.

▶ In Week Two, I asked you to try adding some green or black tea to your diet. I hope you have come to enjoy this healthful beverage and continue to drink it.

▶ Food is the best way to get your antioxidants and thanks to their potent flavonoids, the blueberries I asked you to use as a snack or dessert in Week Four offer you optimal—and delicious—antioxidant protection.

▶ I know you can easily maintain these dietary changes into this week and in the weeks that follow. And once you have mastered one or more of Waldy's sensuous meals, the benefits in terms of health, hardness, and happiness will be innumerable.

Erection Rx

▶ Talk sex with your physician.

One . . . Two . . . Three . . . Foreplay

DAN, age 52—It's not like my remote control

Dan was insistent that I write him a prescription for Levitra. "You have to understand," he said. "She's my second wife. She's much younger and I don't want to let her down like that."

Dan recounted his misadventures from the previous night. "I got into bed after a long, stressful day at work. We have a pending deal and it is taking all of my efforts to keep it on track. When Sarah came to bed, she was on me like a tigress. She wanted some quick sex. Believe me, I am ecstatic when my wife initiates a sexual encounter. While I would never turn down an invitation like that, I was taken by surprise because my thoughts were actually elsewhere.

Meanwhile Back at the Pharmacy . . .

A guy nervously approaches the counter at the local drugstore.

"Excuse me, ma'am," he stammers. "May I speak to the pharmacist?"

"I'm the pharmacist," the woman says. "It's just my sister and me here. What can I do for you?"

"Ah, well, it's rather embarrassing."

"Young man, we've heard everything," she assures him. "Don't be nervous."

"Well, I've had this erection for days, and I can't get rid of it. What can you give me for it?"

"Wait here. I'll be right back," she says, walking into the office. A few minutes later, she stepped back to the counter.

"My sister and I can give you $20,000 cash and 10 percent of the business."

WEEK FOUR   WEEK FIVE   WEEK SIX

"Unfortunately, no matter how hard Sarah tried, I just couldn't get an erection," he said. "That's why I need the Levitra. I don't want to ever discourage my wife and I don't want to let something like this ever happen again."

Dan admitted that he still had regular hard morning erections and whenever he made sexual overtures to Sarah, he never had any hardness problems. These were good healthy signs, I explained to Dan, and reasons why he didn't need Levitra. What Dan had was a temporary libido issue, not a problem with achieving a hard erection.

"As men get older," I said, "foreplay becomes just as important to men as it is to women most of the time. Contrary to what some men and women think, we really don't have an 'on/off' erection switch on the back of our heads. In order for an older man to achieve a hard erection, it becomes necessary to recruit all of the senses to get the erection process into high gear.

"When you were younger, just hearing that a woman wanted to have sex with you was often enough to trigger instantaneous hardness, no matter what the time of day or night, or what particular stressors you had in your life. However, with increasing age, varying degrees of tactile stimulation, smell, and visual stimuli have to come into play in order to recruit the nerve fibers necessary for an erection to occur."

Hearing this, Dan was visibly relieved. He came to understand that the timing had been off when his wife had made her overtures and that no erection drug could have solved that problem. "With just a little more foreplay," I told him, "you'll be good to go."

Here's the rest of the story: Dan originally came in asking for a sample of Levitra and I gave him a prescription for the medication as a "just in case." He never filled it.

The Good News Is, Your Bladder Ailment Has Been Cured . . .

In 2003, a Texas man woke up from bladder surgery to discover that doctors had removed his penis without his permission.

FOREPLAY LESSONS

▶ **Lesson 1**   Men don't come with "on/off" erection switches.

▶ **Lesson 2**   While sexual thoughts are often enough to cause a hard erection in a younger man, other stimuli will be needed as a man ages to achieve the same degree of hardness.

▶ **Lesson 3**   Women have successfully educated men in a woman's need for adequate foreplay—men need to establish the same for themselves. Foreplay is for couples, not a gender.

ANTIOXIDANTS = ANTISOFTNESS

This week I want you to add vitamins C and E to your antioxidant arsenal to help battle free radicals, the unstable molecules that lead to so many of our common diseases. These two vitamins work great together in tandem to produce their antioxidant effect, while protecting each other from oxidation. They also help other antioxidants such as Pycnogenol, resveratrol, and grape seed extract do their good work throughout the body.

Vitamin C Benefits Vitamin C is present in citrus fruits as well as most other fruits and vegetables, including melons, strawberries, red peppers, dark green leafy vegetables, potatoes, and tomatoes. These natural sources of vitamin C can help block the heart-damaging effects of atherosclerosis caused by free radical damage to the basic structure of cells. This powerful antioxidant also increases the permeability as well as the strength of the capillaries and helps lower both cholesterol and fat levels.

66 Erections have enormous implications for a man's partner, both in the emotional and physical shared health of the relationship.

Vitamin E Benefits By mopping up the free radicals, vitamin E, along with C, inhibits the oxidation of LDL cholesterol. This is important because once this "bad" lipoprotein is oxidized it can become trapped in the intima of the artery walls, damaging the lining of the artery and leading to the accumulation of fatty plaque deposits. In addition, vitamin E may help reduce the ability of the blood to clot, thereby lowering heart attack risk. The inflammatory blood vessel process, which has been linked with coronary artery disease, can also be reduced by supplementation with vitamin E.

HOW MEDICINE AND SCIENCE EVOLVE

Medicine and science are always evolving, with new studies being published almost daily on topics ranging from how a particular food can reverse heart disease to how a prescription drug can lower cholesterol. Unfortunately, in reporting these new research findings, the news media often fail to discuss the particular nuances of a study or to describe who the test subjects were, how long the research lasted, or why other similar studies had shown no effect or else very little effect.

There have been innumerable examples of public panic over medical studies. One that comes to mind, however, is a recent vitamin E study in which the media unnecessarily scared people into thinking high supplementation with vitamin E not only did not reduce the risk of early death but actually might increase it.

When it comes to any medical study you may have concerns about, do what I always tell my patients to do: Discuss it with your doctor. A well-informed physician will generally have multiple sources of medical and scientific information as well as a network of colleagues who can provide broader perspective on the merits of the study.

THE HARDNESS FACTOR VITAMIN C AND E PROGRAM

Scientists are just beginning to understand how these nutrients work within the body, but it is becoming eminently clear that a **daily intake** of **vitamins C and E,** either from your daily meals or supplements, plays a major **protective role** within the body.

For **optimal levels of vitamin C,** I recommend at **least 500 mg** of vitamin C daily for maximum antioxidant power and heart and hardness protection. While food is the best source of vitamin C, if you are like most of my patients who barely eat three portions of fruits and vegetables, a daily supplement is definitely in order.

Getting adequate quantities of vitamin E that offer heart and hardness protection from food is often a problem. Most of my patients who adhere to **low-fat diets** have **difficulty** getting the **recommended 200–400 IU of E** from their daily diet. This is because vitamin E is found primarily in high-fat foods such as nuts, seeds, vegetable oils, and mayonnaise. Therefore, the best way for optimal daily vitamin E intake is through a supplement.

When purchasing your vitamins, look for **"natural"** vitamin E supplements containing **"mixed tocopherols."** The synthetic versions of the vitamin contain forms that are poorly utilized by the body. **Take** up to **400 IUs every day with your meal** to ensure optimal absorption.

SENSUAL NUTRITION

Historically, Americans have always celebrated with food. Whether it's the Fourth of July, Thanksgiving, or New Year's Eve, Americans like to prepare favorite recipes to commemorate these special times. Food isn't just for our stomachs, but for our hearts and souls as well. It's now time for you to celebrate your completion of the Hardness Factor Six-Week Program. There is no better way to commemorate this milestone than with this special

Waldy Malouf–inspired celebration menu. It's a meal that Waldy prepared for my beautiful wife, Kiki, and me. Awesome.

If you have been preparing Waldy's sensuous food selections each week of the program, you undoubtedly enhanced your culinary skills. I am also sure that your taste buds are more refined; food tastes different now. You have cut back on saturated fats. You are not drinking alcohol as much. If you smoke cigarettes, hopefully you have found a way to stop. Understanding the impact of too many calories on health and hardness, your portion sizes have shrunk. You now feel better and look better.

For this special occasion, Waldy has designed a sumptuous dinner that is both extraordinary but easy to prepare **(see page 207).** It's a meal that is tasty and rich with flavor, but light enough not to spoil appetites for the big bedroom feasts to come later on. Enjoy!

This Week's Menus

MENU ONE

SWORDFISH STEAKS IN A MUSTARD SEED CRUST

Butter Lettuce Salad with Red Pepper Vinaigrette
Swordfish Steaks in a Mustard Seed Crust
Poached Pears with Apricots and Almonds

MENU TWO

CHICKEN BREAST WITH MUSTARD, ALMONDS, AND THYME

Tuna Carpaccio with Basil and Arugula
Chicken Breast with Mustard, Almonds, and Thyme
Blueberry Cobbler
(See **Appendix II** for recipes)

WEEK ONE   WEEK TWO   WEEK THREE

Diabesity: A Natural Softener

CLIFF, age 22—A walking time bomb

Cliff was in my office a week after he graduated from college. A 22-year-old math genius who was heading to MIT for graduate studies in a little more than two months, he told me that he was totally depleted. The final year of undergraduate work had been a real struggle and he was not sure he could handle the workload at MIT.

Cliff now found himself nodding off during the day. He was forgetful. In addition, it was the periods of dark, gloomy moods that precipitated his recent breakup with his longtime girlfriend. His faulty erections, he admitted, also played a part in his overall grumpy disposition.

A simple blood test confirmed what I had suspected: diabesity, the medical condition of having both Type 2 diabetes (noninsulin dependent) and excessive weight. Cliff carried 228 pounds on his slight six-foot frame, with most of the weight in his bulging belly. Excessive weight around the gut is a clear marker for diabesity. He was virtually sedentary, with his only physical activity coming from walking a few blocks to the local library and moving the mouse on his computer. This inactivity was contributing to his problems.

Cliff's cholesterol was 242, when it should have been well below 200. His elevated blood sugar and insulin levels put him in the early Type 2 diabetes category. Barely out of his teens, he now had the same poor health risk profile as a much older, physically inactive adult male.

If Cliff didn't take any steps to reverse this condition right now, I explained to him, he faced a future of mild erectile dysfunction eventually turning to severe ED. Diabetes damages the blood vessels and the nerves responsible for erections. He was already experiencing weak erections, which was not surprising. Almost 10 percent of men with diabetes who are between the ages of 20 and 29 have hardness problems.

> 66 Research now shows that half of the men with diabetes will experience hardness difficulties as much as fifteen years earlier than men without diabetes. Moreover, as men with diabetes get older, the likelihood of having hardness problems jumps to 70 percent after the age of 55.

Research now shows that half of the men with diabetes will experience hardness difficulties as much as fifteen years earlier than men without diabetes. Moreover, as men with diabetes get older, the likelihood of having hardness problems jumps to 70 percent after the age of 55.

If Cliff's diabesity was allowed to progress, there would be a need for daily medication and regular blood sugar testing. Untreated, the diabesity would lead to heart disease, blindness, and kidney failure. The predicament for Cliff was certainly grim but since we had caught it relatively early there was a good chance that it could be reversed. That is, if Cliff was willing to do what was necessary to radically alter the lifestyle disaster he had inadvertently created for himself.

Since he was already in the throes of a serious medical ailment, I mapped out a more aggressive form of my Hardness Factor program for him. I took out a calendar and set a deadline of two months to bring about significant changes in his lifestyle. In eight weeks I wanted him to adopt a series of modifications that were specifically designed to pare off the dangerous body fat around his waist and the excess weight in general. This would also help reduce his blood sugar and insulin levels, and bring his cholesterol into a safe range. These positive changes would also enhance his hardness. Here's what Cliff agreed to do, effective immediately:

Change his diet—radically. Eliminated from his diet were all forms of junk food and sugary fruit juices that typically made up his daily lunch. These were replaced by plenty of vegetables, whole grains, broiled turkey breast, chicken, and fish. I instructed Cliff to cut down on portion size, too, and eliminate mindless snacking altogether.

And get physical on a daily basis. He was to switch off the TV and head outside, using a step counter to measure his daily hikes around the city. When he called after the first week, he told me he was out exploring Central Park, and taking more than 11,000 steps a day, which was great. His girlfriend, Molly, was now back in his life, and they had joined a local gym. They lifted weights together three days a week under the watchful eyes of a fitness trainer, motivating him even more to succeed with his program.

Cliff was nervous when he came back to my office eight weeks later for his blood work results. He had gone from 27 percent body fat to a much healthier 25 percent. He was able to pull in two notches on his belt and it showed. Most of his 14-pound weight loss seemed to come from around his belly, but he still had a way to go. Better yet, his cholesterol had dropped to 212 and his blood sugar levels were now normal. Three months later, his cholesterol was an outstanding 178.

I congratulated Cliff on his success but also let him know that this was just the beginning of a lifelong commitment to his health. The reward from his eight weeks of hard work was not just a change in his weight and blood work, but the ability to finally take control of his health, integrating a healthy, physically fit body with his masterful mental gifts.

INSULIN LESSONS

Lesson 1   Diabesity patients pose the greatest medical challenge to doctors.

Lesson 2   Patients suffering from diabesity are "walking time bombs" who would benefit from admission to the intensive care unit (ICU) at a local hospital.

Lesson 3   If untreated, men with diabesity will end up in an ICU.

Lesson 4   Young men with diabesity are on an advanced path to progressive vascular disease and ED.

Lesson 5   Young men with diabesity are at a medical crossroads. If lifestyle modifications are adhered to, the condition can be corrected. If not, there will be a rapid decline in health resulting in high blood pressure, arthritis, depression, diabetes, and erectile dysfunction.

ARE YOU AT RISK FOR DIABESITY?

Many of the 16 million Americans who have diabetes aren't even aware of it. That's because, like hypertension and elevated cholesterol, diabetes comes on slowly, without any overt symptoms. A common tip-off for all three of these ailments, however, is decreased hardness. The good news is that like high blood pressure and cholesterol, diabesity can be controlled, and in some cases reversed and prevented, with the same lifestyle measures I outlined for Cliff.

Diabetes is a metabolic disorder characterized by a breakdown in the body's ability to efficiently utilize glucose, the main type of sugar produced when foods are digested. Glucose is needed by all cells in the body for energy. Most cells can absorb adequate glucose only in the presence of insulin, a hormone produced by the pancreas. However, when natural insulin production is curtailed due to overeating and lack of exercise, or when cells don't respond appropriately to the insulin, serious metabolic problems are created.

DIABETES CHECKLIST

Diabetes often goes undiagnosed because many of its symptoms seem so harmless. However, research indicates that the early detection of diabetes symptoms and subsequent treatment can decrease the chance of developing the complications of diabetes.

Check off any symptoms of diabetes you may be experiencing:

1. Frequent Urination
  ○ **Yes**   ○ **No**

2. Excessive thirst
  ○ **Yes**   ○ **No**

3. Extreme hunger
  ○ **Yes**   ○ **No**

4. Unusual weight loss
  ○ **Yes**   ○ **No**

5. Increased fatigue
  ○ **Yes**   ○ **No**

6. Irritability
  ○ **Yes**   ○ **No**

7. Blurry vision
  ○ **Yes**   ○ **No**

NOTE: If you have one or more of these diabetes symptoms, contact your doctor immediately.

DIABETES: WHAT YOU CAN DO

With Americans getting fatter due to overeating and not enough physical activity, the incidence of Type 2 diabetes—and with it, hardness problems—has been rising dramatically, approaching epidemic proportions. Every man should know the symptoms of Type 2 diabetes, which usually develop slowly over the years: faulty erections, excessive thirst, frequent urination, constant hunger, blurred vision, fatigue, and numbness or tingling in the hands and feet.

Everyone age 45 and older should get a blood test for diabetes every three years. The following men, however, need more frequent screening, starting at age 30:

▶ Hispanic
▶ African American
▶ Asian
▶ Native American
▶ Obese
▶ Sedentary
▶ Those with a strong family history of diabetes

ERECTION Rx

When I ask men, "Are you happy with your sex life?" most tell me that it could be better. When I ask them, "Are you happy with your erection hardness?" most don't know that erections are under their control. As I have said so often, while hardness is certainly good, harder is even better. Many of my patients are startled when I first query them. They often will say that their previous doctors never brought up the subject. Moreover, unless they, the patients, had a specific or pressing sexual problem, they didn't mention it, either. That's a problem, since 90 percent of men with hardness problems have never mentioned it to their doctors.

On the other hand, there are men who are very happy that I brought up the subject, using my openness in wanting to help as a chance to unload about intimate subjects that had really been bothering them.

Talking about hardness issues with your doctor is an excellent example of a person taking charge of his health. When you see your doctor, I am sure you aren't shy about discussing your blood pressure or cholesterol, colds or the flu, weight lost or gained. Holding back information about sexual concerns cheats both you and your doctor. For one, the physician won't be able to perform a comprehensive checkup or offer a solution for a solvable problem. Moreover, the patient, of course, will not get the relief that might be readily available.

> 66 Are you happy with your erection? Has it changed? Does it seem different?

Keeping the lines of communication open benefits both patients and their doctors. If you're shy about discussing sex consider this: Altering sexual patterns for the better is often as simple as changing a prescription for a medication already being used. In addition, new and better medical answers are being developed every day. Taking advantage of them means making your life better. Isn't that worth a little initial awkwardness?

SEXUAL FITNESS: MEN NEVER HAD A JANE FONDA

In order for a relationship to truly work, couples need to have a commonality when it comes to central beliefs and interests. They also need a basic physical commonality. If not, a wedge will be created between them.

This is a brief story about Ed, a patient, who had let himself slide physically, while his wife, Emily, continued to work at her fitness. It spotlights another important aspect of the Hardness Factor: the important link between physical and sexual fitness.

ED, age late 50s—Alone on the dance floor

I was at an outdoor cocktail party at the home of a friend one balmy evening this past summer. While drinking a glass of wine, Ed, a contemporary of mine, came over and asked what interesting changes I was witnessing in medicine. Ed was a longtime editor with a major publisher and he had a keen interest in medical topics.

I began detailing some of my ongoing research in male hardness, going over what it meant to be sexually fit, and how much penile hardness is intimately linked with one's level of overall sexual fitness.

"Sexual fitness? I never heard that before," Ed said. "Tell me more."

"Sexual fitness is the overall link between mind, body, and health," I explained. "The more physically fit you are, which entails flexibility, muscular strength, and aerobic capacity, the higher your level of penile hardness, ability, and overall sexual confidence." Ed politely interrupted. "This is really interesting. Hold that thought. My wife has to hear this," he said. He beckoned his wife over, who was an editor of a popular medical newsletter and who had just finished dancing with a young man.

Emily, a stylish woman in her early 50s, with dark, curly hair flecked with some gray highlights, was full of energy. She turned to her husband, cutting him off almost in mid-sentence. "Honey, I am sexually fit. *You're* the problem. Now, do you want to dance with me? Come on."

I found myself in an extremely awkward position as I watched my fitness theory play out right in front of me. Stung by his wife's blunt appraisal, Ed threw his hands up, as if to say, "What am I supposed to do about it?" and sheepishly followed his wife back to the dance area.

It was obvious that Ed was out of touch with the fact that being

> 66 It was obvious that Ed was out of touch with the fact that being sexually fit—fit for sex—was such a powerful issue with his wife, Emily.

WEEK ONE   WEEK TWO   WEEK THREE

sexually fit—fit for sex—was such a powerful issue with Emily. Unfortunately, I don't find this to be very unusual. I have met many attractive and vibrant middle-aged women who stand by—often in annoyance—as their husbands atrophy right in front of them.

Many men just don't understand that their wives are in such great physical shape for beauty, health, and yes, sexual reasons. I call it the "Fonda Effect," a permanent remnant from the very successful Jane Fonda aerobic workout tapes and books from years ago.

Many women continue to take a proactive approach to their sexual identities. They eat sensibly. They exercise regularly. While primed and ready for sex, many have mates who have let themselves go physically, losing their interest in a vital sexual relationship as the excess pounds and body fat have increased. While successful in many other areas of their lives, when it comes to sexual fitness, many men still need to take a cue from women and take positive steps to boost their sexual fitness.

DANCE LESSONS

Lesson 1 A couple may be in the same chronological zone (age) but biologically (how they function) they can be on very different levels due to their attention to important lifestyle issues.

Lesson 2 You don't want to create a chronological/biological gap with your partner.

Lesson 3 If lifestyle changes aren't made, the gap will increase, possibly causing both sexual and interpersonal problems.

Lesson 4 Who has a greater vital force in your relationship— you or your partner? You had better have a vital force equal to or slightly greater than that of your partner.

SIX-WEEK PROGRAM

1. HARDNESS FACTOR

Rate your current level of hardness for Day Forty-two of the program. (Check off one box.)

○ Soft   ○ Soft/Hard   ○ Hard
○ Very Hard   ○ Like a Steel Beam

2. SEXUAL FITNESS

FROM WEEKS 1–5:

- Side Lunge Reach (15 repetitions each leg)
- Angry Cat Stretch (4 times)
- Woodchopper Exercise (20 repetitions)
- Single Leg Bridge NEW
  > Lift into Bridge.
  > Take one foot off the floor and bridge up and down on the single leg, slowly and in balance with abdominals drawn in for 5 repetitions.
  > Return to the floor, lift into Bridge, and repeat with the opposite leg for 5 repetitions.
- Hip-Flexor Stretch (hold for 15 seconds)

1. Neck Stretch NEW

Many men find that their neck stiffens after tilting their heads up while involved in cunnilingus. Here is an effective stretch to remove any resulting aches and pains.

- Place one hand on the back of your head.
- Inhale deeply and, as you exhale, lower your chin to your chest and press *gently* with your hand.
- Hold this position for 5 seconds.
- Inhale deeply as you slowly raise your head back up.
- **Repeat 4 times.**

FROM WEEKS 1–5:

- Classic Push-Ups (3 sets of 10 repetitions)
- Plank (5 sets, hold 60 seconds, rest 15 seconds)
- Cobra (10 repetitions)
- Squat (20 repetitions)
- Squat Thrust (5 repetitions, with Classic Push-Up performed after Thrust while in Push-Up position)
- Single-Leg Squat (5 repetitions each leg without a chair)

2. Back Extension NEW

This will stretch your abdominal area and strengthen the muscles of your lower back.

- Lie face down on the floor, place your hands shoulder-width apart, palms flat on the floor, fingers pointing forward.
- Lift your chest slowly off the floor, exhaling as you lift; keep your pelvis and legs in contact with the floor.
- Pause for 3 seconds at the top of the motion and then slowly return your chest to the floor.
- **Perform 5 repetitions.**

3. Child's Pose

This position is not only relaxing, but it will gently stretch the lower back, chest, and shoulders. Note: Skip this exercise if you have any history of knee problems or experience pain.

- Get on the floor on your hands and knees, with your hands shoulder-width apart, fingers straight ahead.
- Lower your buttocks onto your ankles and your forehead onto the floor. *(Note: If you're uncomfortable letting your weight rest on your lower legs, place a pillow between your buttocks and legs, taking pressure off your knees and allowing you to relax and let your weight drop backward.)*
- Crawl your fingertips forward on the floor as you relax into the stretch. *(Note: If you are not flexible enough through your hips and your upper torso cannot bend so you reach the floor, place a pillow in front of you and let your head and/or your whole upper body rest on it.)*
- **Hold for 60 seconds and relax.**

3. WALKING

Take 10,000 steps a day. Circle each day you achieved this goal:

Sunday   Monday   Tuesday   Wednesday   Thursday   Friday   Saturday

4. HARDNESS FACTOR SUPPLEMENTS

FROM WEEKS 1–5:

Pycnogenol **(80 mg)**/L-arginine **(3 g)** mixture or Pycnogenol Plus or Prelox Blue.

2 horny goat weed capsules.

2 Omega-3 fatty acid capsules.

Red wine **(200 mg)** and grape seed extract **(100mg)** daily.

2 400-mg no-flush niacin pills if your HDL level is in a good range. Speak to your doctor about higher doses if HDL levels are low.

Vitamins C and E `NEW`
500 mg of vitamin C and 200–400 IU of vitamin E.

5. SENSUAL NUTRITION

Prepare three sensuous meals this week.
- Swordfish Steaks in a Mustard Seed Crust
- Chicken Breast with Mustard, Almonds, and Thyme
- Grand Feast

A MAN @ 65

Hardness is wavering in all but those who have worked over the decades to enhance and maintain hardness.

The refractory period may stretch to a day for many men.

The impact of untreated atherosclerosis, diabetes, hypertension, and unhealthy lifestyle choices makes erections iffy and problematic for many men.

Medication is needed by many men to achieve an erection.

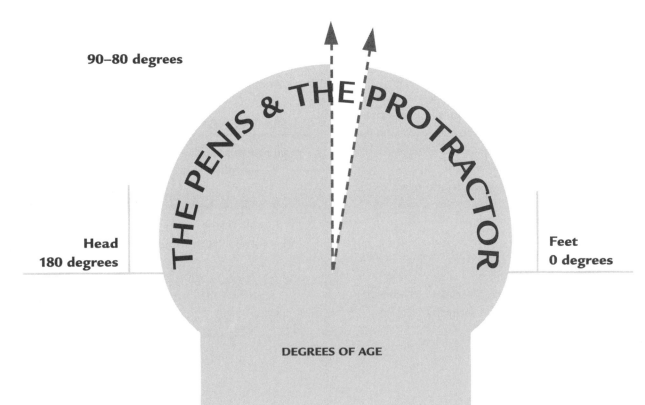

90–80 degrees

THE PENIS & THE PROTRACTOR

Head
180 degrees

Feet
0 degrees

DEGREES OF AGE

THE LAST WEEK—HARD IS GREAT

You have completed the six weeks of the Hardness Factor Program. Do you realize just how much you have accomplished in only forty-two days? You have enhanced your hardness, which is great. But more important, you have improved your health profile and set yourself firmly on the pathway to optimal health. You are now effectively empowered to realize your full potential and alter the course of your life. You deserve all the credit. It's all about men taking care of their health. Welcome to the club.

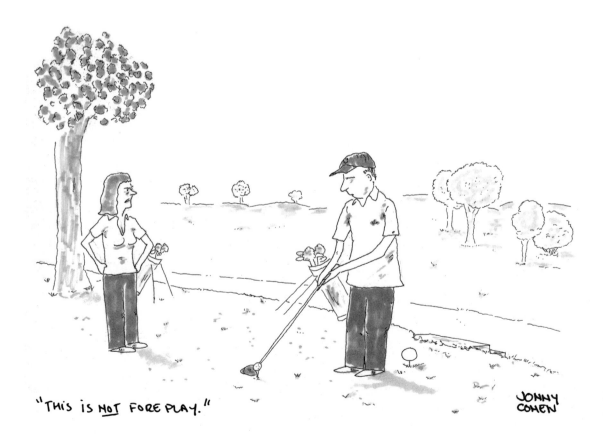

"THIS IS NOT FORE PLAY."

Part Three

HARDNESS FOR LIFE

(or at Least Through Friday Night)

OPEN ONLY IN CASE OF
EMERGENCY

THE HARDNESS FACTOR
FOUR-DAY INSURANCE POLICY*

- Enhances hardness in only four days
- A quick, effective lifestyle program
- Sensitizes blood vessels and nerve endings
- Combats vascular disease
- Increases libido
- Bolsters confidence

NOTE: This is an abbreviated, intense program recommended for emergency use only. There is nothing in this chapter that is not found in the Hardness Factor Six-Week Program.

* To be opened only in an emergency.

10

THE HARDNESS FACTOR

FOUR-DAY INSURANCE POLICY>>>>>>>>

The big date is coming up and you want to be ready for everything and anything. Nevertheless, you have your doubts. Your performance anxiety has some basis in fact, since your hardness waned at the wrong time, leaving you staring at the ceiling trying to explain what went wrong with the hydraulics. You don't have six weeks—your date is Saturday night!

LESS THAN A WEEK AWAY

What are you to do now? The weekend is approaching, you don't have time for the Six-Week Program, and you have to step up to the plate again. Do you have to rely on one of the prescription erection drugs? Well, you can certainly go that route if you are truly desperate.

SEND HELP FAST

But I have a much better way for ensuring and maximizing hardness for the man in a hurry. When you need immediate assistance, I have just the "pick-me-up" that a man needs to stay on the playing field. I call it the Hardness Factor Insurance Policy.

The hardness of his penis is the last thing a man needs to worry about in an ongoing relationship or while traveling the dating circuit. Let him worry instead about romance, intimacy, and fun. The beauty of the Hardness Factor Four-Day Insurance Policy is that it helps take the worry out of erections. Follow my hardness suggestions for four days and it will help eliminate self-doubt and minimize physical deterrents by enhancing the all-important oxygenation capability of the heart and penile tissues. This in turn will strengthen erections. Libido will be increased as well, much to the surprise of men and their partners.

If you are that man in a hurry, I want to outline the Insurance Policy and describe exactly what I want you to do over the next four days. This brief but highly effective program is tailored so you will be better prepared for optimal sex by the end of the fourth day.

STEP ONE

SENSUAL NUTRITION: MAKE CHANGES IN WHAT YOU EAT

In the last two decades, the correlation between nutrition and optimal performance has become better understood. Guess what? Your sexual performance is greatly impacted by exactly what and how much you consume. Here's what you need to do:

Cut back on portion size. Try to eat 10 percent less at each meal. Scaling back on calories will leave you sated but not stuffed. By Day Four, you may notice the loss of a pound or two on your scale. That is important because the amount of fat in your gut affects the amount of testosterone available to you—the more fat, the less testosterone.

Avoid fatty foods. Stop shocking your blood vessels. Fatty, high-calorie foods may taste great, but they are not kind to erections. The fats injure your blood vessels to the point where they are stunned, preventing them from being totally responsive when sexual signals are being transmitted from brain to penis. Penile nerves lose their sensitivity when cholesterol builds up. Since dietary cholesterol comes mainly from animal sources, you need to recognize and avoid it. Top saturated fat culprits include egg yolks, butter, cream, fatty red meats, and a variety of oils, especially those made from palm and coconut.

Eat plenty of fruits and vegetables. Think five to nine servings every day. This helps lower cholesterol levels, combats cardiovascular disease, and improves blood flow to the penis. These foods also supply many key nutrients. Leafy green vegetables are excellent sources of folic acid, calcium, magnesium, and zinc. Fresh citrus fruits offer plenty of vitamin C.

Spice up your foods. Spices like chili and ginger can contribute to sexual pleasure and performance.

Prepare your training meals. The expression "You are what you eat" takes on a completely new meaning when men follow the suggested four-day meal plans I worked out with Chef Waldy Malouf and nutritionist Tana Kokol. The key to their recommendations is that they keep the saturated fats down, with enough calories to give you the necessary energy to carry out your daily tasks.

As you will see, they have added a variety of spices to many of their meal selections to expose you, your palate, and your dinner guest to new taste sensations. On Day Four, you are ready to step out, transformed and revitalized. The ultimate date dinner recommended by Waldy offers a host of luscious textures and sensuous flavors designed to excite and create the mood for sexual intimacy.

Here are complete menus for four days of Hardness Nutrition.

DAY 1 Tuesday

BREAKFAST

1 bowl oatmeal *(soluble fiber lowers LDL cholesterol)*

1 cup skim or 1% lowfat milk

1 banana

1 handful blueberries *(they're the highest in antioxidants)*

1 cup tea *(powerful antioxidant properties)*

MIDMORNING SNACK

1 small handful mixed almonds and golden raisins

LUNCH

1 whole grain pita

3 tablespoons hummus

1 sliced tomato

Alfalfa sprouts

Romaine lettuce

Sprinkling of Feta cheese

½ onion, sliced

1 serving three bean salad (kidney, green, and garbanzo beans in a vinaigrette dressing: 2 tablespoons extra-virgin olive oil, 1 teaspoon balsamic vinegar)

1 cup black or green tea

MIDAFTERNOON SNACK

1 bowl blueberries

DINNER

Miso soup

2 rolls *(extra sesame seeds on the rolls)*

3 pieces sashimi *(no rolls or sushi)*

Mixed green salad with vinaigrette dressing

1 cup green tea

1 cup raspberry sorbet

DAY 2 Wednesday

BREAKFAST

1 cup 1% cottage cheese

1 handful raisins and sunflower seed mix

2–3 whole grain crackers *(Kavli Crackers or Finn Crisp)*

1 apple or pear

1 cup tea

MIDMORNING SNACK

1 high protein energy bar *(Luna or other)*

LUNCH

8 steamed crab dumplings with dipping sauce on the side

1 cup lightly sautéed vegetables with garlic sauce on the side

1 cup brown rice *(an amount a little smaller than your fist)*

1 cup black tea

MIDAFTERNOON SNACK

2 Mini Babybels *(small rounds of lowfat Gouda cheese)*

1 handful grape tomatoes

DINNER

1 bowl gazpacho

3–4 ounces broiled salmon

Broccoli rabe sautéed with garlic and olive oil

1 baked sweet potato

1 cup fresh berry parfait made with nonfat topping

FOUR-DAY INSURANCE POLICY MENU

DAY 3 Thursday

BREAKFAST

Scrambled eggs with mushrooms, onions, and herbs *(made with two egg whites and one whole egg in a nonstick pan)*

1–2 slices whole grain bread

1 tablespoon all-fruit preserves

1 cup tea

MIDMORNING SNACK

Sliced apple

1 tablespoon peanut butter *(or other nut butter)*

LUNCH

1 large vegetable salad with romaine lettuce

3 ounces tuna

Tomatoes, kidney beans, onion, peppers, olives, carrots, celery

Extra-virgin olive oil dressing

8-ounce juice spritzer (juice and seltzer with ice and lime: ½ fruit juice and ½ seltzer)

MIDAFTERNOON SNACK

Fresh fruit smoothie (fresh fruit, 8 oz. fruit juice, ice, nonfat yogurt, two ice cubes blended together)

DINNER

4 ounce steak

1 cup lightly sautéed green beans and slivered almonds

3–4 boiled new potatoes, skin seasoned with parsley

Tomato and onion salad vinaigrette

1 glass red wine

DAY 4 Friday

BREAKFAST

1 cup fruit salad (cut up apples, pineapples, blueberries, strawberries, and melon)

6–8 ounces nonfat yogurt

1 small whole-grain nut roll

1 cup tea or coffee

MIDMORNING SNACK

4 crystallized chewy ginger candies

LUNCH

White meat turkey club sandwich on whole grain bread

3 ounces fresh turkey breast, one slice Canadian bacon, tomato, lettuce, low-fat mayo

Ginger beer

MIDAFTERNOON SNACK

1 cup grapes

A Hardness-Friendly Dinner Date

It's date night and you are at the restaurant. A little nervous? Most likely. Your first instinct may be to order a drink or two to get in the mood. Danger! The reason you turned to this chapter is because you are concerned about what might be happening later on. Limit your drinking. Every sip you take will impact your sexual chemistry.

You have prepared your mind and body over the course of four days. Don't let the restaurant menu be a minefield ready to do you in. The point of this meal is to have an enjoyable time with your companion, while keeping your penis sensitive and awake. Choose the wrong appetizer or entrée, and all that cream, butter, fat, and alcohol will shock your endothelium (blood vessel lining) and put your penis to sleep. You will suffer a brain-penis disconnect.

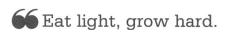 Eat light, grow hard.

While your brain may be conjuring up thoughts sexual, your penis will never get the complete message if it is put into this "nap" state. No matter how many cups of coffee you drink later, if you have inadvertently put your penis to sleep, it's not going to fully awaken. Therefore, eat light, grow hard.

Look at this dinner as a training meal. You are getting ready to perform later. This meal is only helping to set the mood and give you enough calories for some upcoming physical fun.

Here are some important guidelines:

- Avoid all high-fat foods. This includes braised, basted, escalloped, sautéed, creamy, and fried selections.
- Choose entrées that are steamed, broiled, baked, poached, grilled, or roasted.
- Take a pass on all foods high in MSG or salt.
- Think light. Split your entrée with your partner.
- Have salad dressing served on the side. Better yet, opt for vinegar and oil.
- Trim the fat from red meat and have any poultry dish served without the skin.
- Choose fruit or sherbet for dessert.

> **And if you stay home try this (this is also the**
> **Six Week Celebration meal—so you are sort of cheating):**
>
> *⁓ Rose Champagne ⁓*
>
> Osetra Caviar with Brioche Toast Points,
> Créme Fraîche, and Chives
> Roasted Oysters with Shallots
> Lamb Chops with Mint and Garlic Relish
> Roasted Carrots with Honey and Black Pepper
> Individual Warm Chocolate Cakes with Roasted Apricots,
> Fresh Cherries, and Seedless Red Grapes
>
> *Green Tea with Honey and Lemon*

STEP TWO

SUPPLEMENT YOUR HARDNESS

Which of nature's legendary hardness enhancers really work? My study results, and those of others, have proven that there are several interesting supplements that significantly enhance hardness and increase sexual interest. There are several important herbal supplements that I want you to take over the next four days.

Pycnogenol/L-arginine I want you to take a special combination of Pycnogenol and L-arginine capsules daily. Purchase a bottle of Pycnogenol and another of L-arginine. **I want you to take 80 milligrams of Pycnogenol and 3 grams of L-arginine every day. You can take 1 Prelox Blue or Pycnogenol Plus capsule, which contains Pycnogenol and L-arginine.**

See the Hardness Factor Shopping List (**pages 325–28**) for some recommended supplements.

Horny Goat Weed: The Great Libido Booster While the Prelox will take care of blood vessels—boosting hardness by maximizing oxygenation—I also want you to buy a bottle of horny goat weed capsules to maximize libido—your sexual appetite. This herb from China boosts sexual interest significantly. Horny goat weed, which has centuries of male satisfaction behind it, is available at health food stores nationwide.

I want you to take 2 capsules twice daily, with an additional 4 capsules two hours before a sexual encounter. In my studies, I have used the Pinnacle brand of horny goat weed called Exotica.

Omega-3s: Vascular Support and Protection Supplementing the daily diet with omega-3 fatty acids commonly found in marine fish oils is one of the important keys to hardness. Scientists have long been singing the praises of omega-3s, and for good reason. Research has shown that the oil reduces the chance of sudden death from heart attack, probably by preventing fatal rhythm disturbances.

I like the fact that these omega-3s, now conveniently available in capsule form, are excellent for reducing levels of triglycerides—another form of fat circulating in your blood—and help protect the blood vessels, including the tiny blood vessels of the penis.

There are many omega-3 products currently available. I have the most experience with ResQ-1250 marine fish oils and recommend them to my patients. **I want you to take 3 grams of omega-3s daily.**

See the Hardness Factor Shopping List **(page 327)** for some recommended omega-3 supplements.

OPCs and Improved Blood Flow For extra protection against insults to blood vessels and enhanced blood flow, add red wine extract and grape seed extract to your four-day regimen. These oligomeric proanthocyanidins (OPCs) enhance the activity of vitamins C and E.

Take 25 milligrams of red wine extract and 100 milligrams of grape seed extract. I use Isotonix OPC-3, a natural food supplement

made up of a combination of grape seed, red wine, and pine bark extracts.

See the Hardness Factor Shopping List **(page 327)** for some recommended OPC supplements.

Vitamins C and E: Overall Antioxidant Protection Based on very impressive laboratory results, I also recommend daily supplementation with 500 milligrams of vitamin C and 200 to 400 IUs of vitamin E, because it is generally very difficult to get such high levels of these important vitamins from food sources. These potent antioxidants seem to protect against heart disease and other conditions, and I believe this will translate to extraordinary endothelial (lining of the veins) protection as well.

HARDNESS FACTOR SUPPLEMENTS

Day One Through Day Four

MORNING
2 horny goat weed capsules
1 Pycnogenol/L-arginine tablet
3 omega-3 fish oil capsules (3 g)
100 mg grape seed extract
50 mg red wine extract
400 IU vitamin E
500 mg vitamin C

EVENING
2 horny goat weed capsules

CAUTION: As with any new medical regimen, it is always best to first review the program with your physician.

STEP THREE

SEXUAL FITNESS FOR HARDNESS

Don't convince yourself otherwise. You are not in the best physical shape possible. Like most Americans, you know that you should be more physically active and that you probably would like to be. You just aren't.

It's time to make some quick yet doable changes over the next four days. Start by standing buck naked in front of a full-length mirror. Take a good, self-critical look. Now, jump up and down twice. Love handles. Bulging gut. Droopy pecs. Rounded shoulders. Flab. Real nice.

Yes, you need to get your muscles in shape for sex. The surest way to enhance hardness, whet sexual appetite, and increase sexual activity is through regular physical activity, something I have found that many of my patients have not really done since PE class in high school. Here's what being in good physical shape will do for you:

- Enhance all the ingredients for passion
- Increase strength and endurance in and out of the bedroom
- Boost self-esteem

Become Strong, Flexible, and Hard. At the most basic level, it is well known that regular exercise improves overall physical fitness and that sexual functioning is an important part of that condition. Exercise also positively affects brain wave activity, which makes you feel energized. Working out regularly builds stamina, preventing or delaying fatigue during sex.

Finally, exercise boosts testosterone levels, leading to heightened libido. As for enhanced body image, regular physical activity will trim away dangerous abdominal fat, the loss of which can positively alter your attitudes about taking your clothes off and having sex.

Perform sexual fitness exercises, such as push-ups, woodchoppers, and squats, and you augment muscle strength and flexibility. This helps to heighten sexual response, a definite asset since orgasm requires considerable muscle activity.

Start Walking for Hardness. One of the surest ways to enhance sexual fitness and overall hardness is through a simple and basic activity—walking. A walking program can rev up hormones, flush stress, whittle away fat, and rejuvenate the body, filling men with renewed vigor, greater confidence, and the glow of good health.

I recommend that you purchase a step counter at your local sporting goods store. This simple measuring device for calculating how far you walk costs about $25. I want you to aim for 5,000 steps a day. That's every day for four days. This is the equivalent of walking about two miles. While it may not seem like much, the payback will be considerable.

Stretching Your Limits. To promote optimal flexibility—the ability to use muscles and joints through their full range of motion—I want you to perform three specific stretches every day. Regular stretching will help to relieve stress, a major contributing factor to hardness problems. When performed in a slow and focused way, stretching can be excellent relaxation therapy as well as a tension easer.

The three stretches described on the following pages will help keep the muscles used during sex limber and flexible and help facilitate a pleasurable sexual experience. Each stretch can be performed in the bedroom on a mat or nonslip carpet placed on the floor. Wear either loose clothing or nothing at all.

DAY ONE Through DAY FOUR

AM & PM

Perform all three stretches

1. **Side Lunge Reach** A great total-body stretch and strengthening exercise for the adductor (inner thigh), abductor (hip area and outer thigh), core, lower back, quadriceps, buttocks, and hamstrings.

   - Stand erect with feet slightly apart, toes pointed forward.
   - Contract your abdominal muscles.
   - Keeping your right leg straight, take a large step sideways with your left foot, toes pointing forward.
   - Bend your left knee.
   - As you lunge to the side, bend your torso over and toward your left thigh.
   - Reach down and touch your left foot with both hands.
   - Return to the start position by pushing off your left foot to straighten your leg.
   - Repeat the exercise with your opposite leg.
   - Perform 10 times with each leg, alternating legs with each repetition.

2. **Hip-Flexor Stretch** Most people have tight hip flexors, so this will enhance flexibility, help prevent back discomfort, test balance, and improve core stability.

   - Stand erect, feet together, hands at your sides.
   - Take a step forward with your right foot, bending your right knee until your left knee is touching the floor.
   - Contract your abdominal muscles and lean forward to gently stretch the front of the left hip flexor.

- ❱ Hold the stretch for 15 seconds.
- ❱ Repeat with the opposite leg.

3. Angry Cat Stretch This exercise actively stretches your lower back.

- ❱ Get on the floor on your hands and knees, with your hands shoulder-width apart, fingers pointing straight ahead.
- ❱ Tuck your chin in toward your chest, contract your abdominal muscles, and round your back up toward the ceiling. Make sure your back is curved, starting at the base of your skull to your tailbone.
- ❱ Hold the rounded back position for 10 seconds.
- ❱ Relax your muscles and return to the start position.
- ❱ **Repeat 3 times.**

FOUR SEXUAL FITNESS EXERCISES

Muscle fatigue during sex is often an unwanted presence. Push-ups, wood-choppers, squats, and cobras can easily take care of that. These are four beneficial exercises to add to the four-day routine because they strengthen and stretch the shoulders, chest, abdominals, buttocks, and legs, all of which are utilized during sexual activity.

Keeping these muscles strong—by using only your body weight for resistance—helps increase strength and stamina, adding to prolonged, more pleasurable sex. In the end, these are the basic exercises that will help change the way that you feel and move for the rest of your life.

DAY ONE Through DAY FOUR

AM	PM
Cobra	Woodchoppers
Push-Ups	Squat

1. **Cobra** This Yoga gem is the best stretching/strengthening combo exercise because it relaxes the muscles of the lower back as it gently stretches the muscles of the abdomen, hips, and neck.

   ▶ Lie on your stomach with your face almost touching the floor.
   ▶ Place your palms on the floor, at the sides of your shoulders.
   ▶ Keep your legs together and the tops of your feet resting on the floor.
   ▶ Push up, bringing your head off the floor.
   ▶ Keep your pelvis pushed into the floor while relaxing the buttocks as best you can.
   ▶ Slowly arch your spine backward, straightening your elbows.
   ▶ Bring your head back and look at the ceiling.
   ▶ Hold the position for 1 second.
   ▶ Descend slowly to the floor and then **repeat 10 times.**

2. **Classic Push-Up** This exercise can quickly strengthen your shoulders, arms, and chest. In addition, using only your body weight, push-ups work your abdominal and back muscles.

   ▶ Lie facedown on the floor with your legs together.
   ▶ Keep your hands at the sides of your chest, palms flat on the floor.
   ▶ Raise your body onto your hands and toes.
   ▶ Inhale and bend your elbows as you slowly lower your body to within 3 inches of the floor.
   ▶ Pause for 1 second.

- Push back up to the starting position.
- **Repeat 3 sets of at least 5 push-ups with a 1-minute rest period between sets.**

3. Woodchopper The Woodchopper is a total body warm-up for the muscles of the upper and lower body, including the chest, back, shoulders, core, and legs.

- Stand with your feet shoulder-width apart, raise your arms up, stretching toward the ceiling with your abdominals drawn in toward your spine.
- Bend your knees while keeping your chest lifted and swing both of your arms between your legs as if you are chopping wood.
- **Repeat 10 times.**

4. Squat The Squat, the undisputed "king of all resistance exercises," will strengthen your buttocks, hamstrings, and quadriceps, as well as the core muscles of your abdomen and chest.

- Stand with your arms fully extended in front of you and your feet hip-width apart.
- Keep your back straight and your weight firmly over your heels.
- Slowly lower your body as if you were going to sit in a chair, until the tops of your thighs are parallel to the floor.
- Pause for 1 second.
- Slowly rise up to standing position.
- **Repeat 10 times.**

WARNING

When you complete this four-day program, you will certainly feel different. You will achieve measurable changes in flexibility, strength, and hardness. Nevertheless, remember that while these changes may seem extraordinary, this abbreviated hardness workout is just a glimpse of what the complete Hardness Factor Six-Week Program offers.

The Hardness Factor Four-Day Insurance Policy is an emergency solution, but it is certainly not the answer for a lifetime of optimal hardness and health. Hardness is a lifestyle, not ninety-six hours' worth of changes in how you live your life. The idea of hardness is to feel good about yourself emotionally and physically. It's a lifestyle decision.

When you have tried this four-day plan and found how well it works, why not feel confident in your abilities and optimal health all the time? As I tell all who participate in the Hardness Factor Program, hard is good, but harder is better. I don't think a commitment of forty-two days is too much to ask in exchange for a lifetime of hardness. I hope that you will now go back to Week One of the Six-Week Program and follow it through to completion.

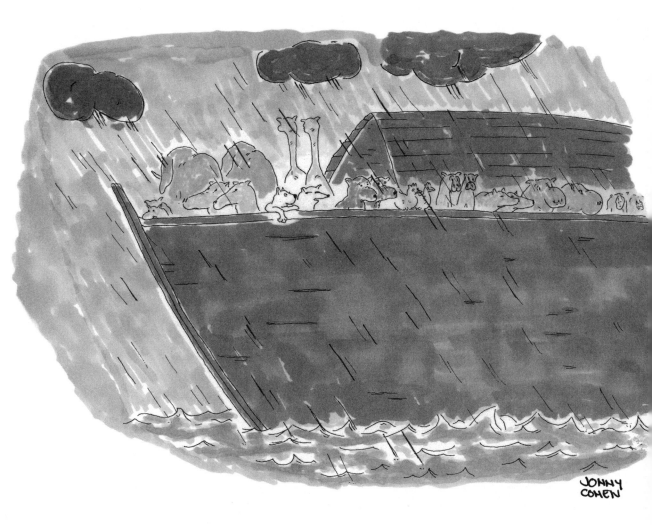

"I HATE THESE SWINGERS PARTIES."

66 *Now, we can do this the hard way or . . . well, actually, there's just the hard way.*

Buffy the Vampire Slayer

11

HARDNESS:
A NEW BAROMETER
OF YOUR HEALTH

According to findings from the landmark Massachusetts Male Aging Study of 1994, a 50-year-old man has a 50/50 chance of having a hardness problem when he awakens in the morning. While this often comes as a shock to many, there are several well-established medical reasons for this, but it doesn't have to be your reality.

YOUR PENIS AGES, TOO

As an internal medicine specialist, I treat men with a variety of medical complaints, many of which affect hardness. I have noted six specific hardness factors that can affect a man's ability to have a firm erection. Outlined below are their primary causes and the Hardness Factor effective solutions for each of them.

HARDNESS CHALLENGE ONE: IMPACT OF AGING

When you were a teenager, an erection would appear just by thinking about, well, just by thinking. Most men have embarrassing stories of erections occurring at the wrong time and the wrong place—such as sitting on a crowded bus and having to stand and get off at the next stop. But the passage of time has a way of changing things for all parts of the body, including the penis.

HARDNESS FACTOR
Self-Preservation

The 51-year-old recently divorced contractor had DIR readings of 989 and 1,298 **(DIR Avg. 1,143)** which were excellent. Interested in preservation and enhancement of his hardness, he also admitted needing to remain hard while using condoms in his new sexual life. After completing the Six-Week Program, his DIR readings went to 1,420 and 1,600 **(DIR. Avg. 1,510),** helping him achieve all of his goals.

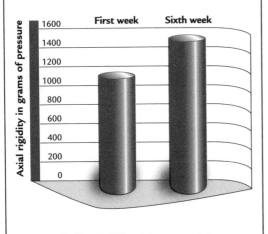

Patient #13 • 51 years old

At 21, putting a condom on is never a problem, for the penis is literally hard as steel. It throbs and even points upward when fully erect. By 40, it is a different story for many. Yes, the penis is still hard, but certainly not like it was twenty years earlier. Over time, a man loses some of his Hardness Factor as nerve connections deteriorate. The penis may now point slightly downward or to the side. For some, it takes more than a hint or a sexual fantasy to develop a full erection.

Testosterone levels start to decline slightly in the 40s and the arousal system now needs more help. By 40 or 50, putting a condom on may actually cause a man to lose his erection. Direct touch to the skin of the penis may be required, so the partner has to take the lead here or provide more caressing of the penis during lovemaking. Ejaculations also take longer and are beginning to lose their power. The refractory period, the time between ejaculations, begins to stretch to twenty minutes or more.

In addition to lower testosterone levels,

growth hormone and the related hormone, DHEA, also begin to drop. With them go a man's sex drive, replaced by more erection problems, an increase in body fat and weight, depression, mood swings, decreased muscle strength, and oftentimes a general decrease in well-being and health.

1. HARDNESS FACTOR SOLUTION

Problems with hardness, although common as a man ages, are not inevitable, nor are they a natural part of aging. Erections may certainly start to lose their hardness as a man gets older, and many men do not get past half-mast by the time they are 50. The fact is, if you want a great sex life at 35, 40, 50, and beyond, you can still have it. Physical changes that have a major impact on sexual performance are typically related to lifestyle issues—and these can all be addressed: the sooner, the better. The best way to ensure a robust sex life in your 50s and 60s is to learn how to increase your hardness in your 30s and 40s.

Awareness of these issues—as well as ones that affect your partner, such as vaginal dryness—will enable a man to maximize his pleasure. If a man develops consistent hardness problems, there may be an underlying disease process of some kind at fault. The good news, however, is that with the Hardness Factor Six-Week Program, these problems are generally reversible through lifestyle changes and supplementation. For those with more advanced disease, there are always the prescription erection medications to boost hardness.

> ### HARDNESS FACTOR
> No More Withdrawals
>
> The 47-year-old banker was in a long-time, stable marriage. With his two children now out of the house, he felt that he needed a boost in his hardness as he and his wife began a new phase in their lives. After six weeks on the program, baseline DIRs of 560, 679, and 900 (**DIR Avg. 713**) went to 1,056, 1,115, and 1,238 (**DIR Avg. 1,286**). In addition, he lost 9 pounds, pulled in his belt two notches, and rejuvenated his sex life significantly. "I miss the kids but it's nice to be noisy again," he said following his six-week checkup.

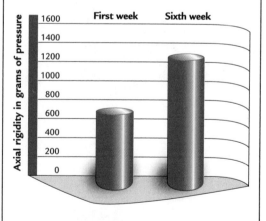

Patient #D-23 • 47 years old

HARDNESS FACTOR
Legal Problems

The 24-year-old law student, under the stress of his ongoing legal studies, part-time job, and poor sleep habits, noted that he was not maximally hard as before and his libido was waning. Initial DIR readings of 710, 695, and 790 (**DIR Avg. 732**) were surprisingly low for such a young man; I expected at least 1,500 grams of pressure or higher.

I explained that he couldn't just expect to "turn on" and be ready for sex but actually had to be physically prepared. Six weeks with the Hardness Factor Program, along with adjustments in his sleep habits, and he had DIR readings of 1,627, 1,745, and 1,810 (**DIR Avg. 1725**).

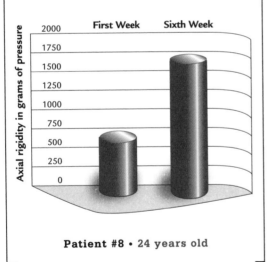

Patient #8 · 24 years old

HARDNESS CHALLENGE TWO: STRESS CAN KEEP YOU DOWN

Stress is everywhere in our lives, and its impact on a man's sex life is quantifiable. Getting the career on track, the daily work grind, shopping, food preparation, travel, a new job, family, a new baby, and the illness or death of a parent or loved one tend to put a damper on a man's ability to have—or want—sex.

When stress starts to take over, a physical response occurs: normal hormonal release is slowed, which eventually impacts testosterone, the master male hormone. Even the heartiest of sexual appetites can become deflated. Blood flow also slows, and that means less blood to flow into the specialized chambers in the penis, which depend on blood for erections.

Unfortunately, life cannot exist without stress. Distress is manifested in sexual, sleeping, or eating issues. That's when it's time to go to the doctor. Nearly all of my patients complain about stress levels and the deep concerns they have about stress's impact on their sex lives.

2. HARDNESS FACTOR SOLUTION

Just thirty minutes of daily exercise triggers a variety of hormones that relax the body and boost the immune system—and this helps lower stress levels considerably. In addition, you need to find ways to put stress in its proper place. Not all problems are of equal weight, and figuring out which situation is really worth worrying about helps to put things in perspective. It comes down to this: In order to limit the effects of stress, focus more on the various solution possibilities, rather than the problem itself. If it can be readily fixed or helped, it is usually not worth the negative hardness and health implications, or the mental energy needed to deal with the so-called problem.

HARDNESS CHALLENGE THREE: SLEEP APNEA ERASES ERECTIONS

Sleep apnea is a common respiratory disorder that affects 4 to 9 percent of adult males. Its most common manifestation is loud snoring and interrupted breathing as he literally gasps for breath when his air passages close off. These mini-choking sessions can occur several hundred times a night, resulting in sleep problems and excessive daytime sleepiness.

The typical patient is an overweight, middle-aged man. Large neck size is a risk factor; sufferers tend to have a collar size larger than 16.5 inches. Excessive alcohol consumption and chronic use of sleeping pills can compound the problem.

3. HARDNESS FACTOR SOLUTION

What man can think of sex when he is so fatigued from lack of sleep triggered by apnea? Dramatic improvement can result from a 10 percent weight loss. Avoiding alcohol and sleeping pills—which relax the dilator throat muscles and cause them to flop on the windpipe—can also help reduce the number of apneic incidents. Eliminating smoking and controlling allergies, both of which inflame throat tissues and cause them to swell, can also help.

Help may be hard to find as too few physicians are aware of the problem, its magnitude, and its treatment. If you suspect sleep apnea, start with your family physician, who will most likely refer you to a pulmonologist, a doctor specializing in respiratory disorders.

HARDNESS CHALLENGE FOUR: EXCESSIVE DRINKING MAKES ERECTIONS SOFT

For most men, moderate drinking of beer, wine, or spirits (one to two drinks per day) is not associated with any health or erection problems. For many, it loosens inhibition. However, when alcohol is consumed in excess—more than three drinks—it acts as a toxic drug with pronounced short- and long-term consequences on arousal and erectile function. (A bottle of 4.5 percent beer, a 4-ounce glass of 12 percent wine, and 1.5 ounces of 80-proof spirits are each considered one drink.)

Steady drinking can inhibit both erection and orgasm. It does so by affecting the production of nitric oxide molecules, which, in turn, makes it difficult for the tissue of the corpus cavernosa to relax enough to allow blood to flow in the penis. If drinking continues over time and alcoholism develops, there is even more damage. The peripheral nervous system is often injured, permanently affecting the ability to have an erection.

HARDNESS FACTOR
Smokes a Downer

The 30-year-old three-pack-a-day smoker had serious hardness problems. DIR readings of 280, 460, and 480 **(DIR Avg. 406)** hammered home the point that he needed to stop smoking, which he did shortly before beginning the program. Six weeks into the program (he was committed to continuing it year round) his DIR readings topped out at 550 grams of pressure **(DIR Avg. 550).** Although this hardness was still well below what it should be for a man his age, it was a nice jump from his previous sub-par efforts and encouraged him to continue with the program.

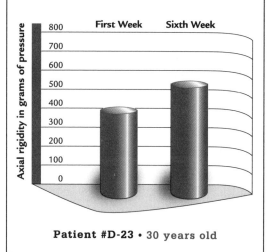

Patient #D-23 • 30 years old

Even worse, heavy drinking is often combined with some variation of the following: steady smoking, overeating, lack of exercise, and drug abuse. This lethal combination nearly always adds to the potential development of severe erection difficulties, or at the very least a softer profile.

> **❝** Steady drinking can inhibit both erection and orgasm— it's enough to drive a man to drink.

4. HARDNESS FACTOR SOLUTION

If ever there were a double-edged sword, it is alcohol. Alcoholic beverages can enhance just as well as ravage, so if you happen to drink, it is best to do so in moderation. In the United States, abuse of alcohol is linked with more than 100,000 deaths a year from disease (liver, lung, and heart ailments as well as increased risk of cerebral hemorrhage) and injury (especially from impaired driving due to alcohol's impact on reaction time and judgment), costing nearly $100 billion in lost worker productivity and health care expenses.

The only solution is to cut down or eliminate drinking. Remember, too, that the sexual consequences of heavy drinking over time include increased estrogen levels (causing feminine characteristics in men, like loss of body hair and muscle mass), shrinking testicles, swollen breasts, and decreased sexual desire and potency.

One mistaken belief is that alcohol is a stimulant and can increase one's sexual performance. In fact, alcohol is a central nervous system depressant and dampens sexual arousal. It also numbs the nerve endings in the penis, leading to a decrease in both the intensity and pleasure in orgasm. In other words, your penis will pass out before you do.

*S*top Picking on the *Little People*

In 2003, a Canadian man was arrested for making death threats against employees of a company he believed was sending him penis enlargement spam in his email.

HARDNESS FACTOR
Four-Day Insurance Policy

A 36-year-old male had hypertension but was not taking any medications. There was a slight change in penile axial rigidity (baseline 900; with the 4-day program 1,038), he felt more confident, and noted that it was easier to sustain an erection. Subject noted the return of "super-hard morning erections" that surprised both him and his wife.

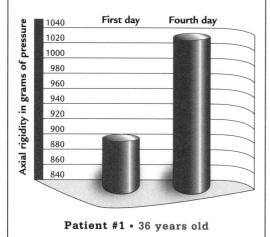

Patient #1 • 36 years old

HARDNESS CHALLENGE FIVE: DRUGS PREVENT HARD ERECTIONS

Cocaine, marijuana, LSD, amphetamines, and barbiturates all have a negative impact on sexual performance, including the capacity to get and keep a hard erection. Many times, hardness problems develop as a side effect of taking a prescription medication. The most common offenders are drugs for high blood pressure, heart ailments, and allergies. Medications used to combat depression, especially the selective serotonin reuptake inhibitors (SSRIs) such as Prozac, Zoloft, and Paxil, can also be the culprits.

Frequently, if a man is taking more than one medication, the damaging effects are cumulative. For example, I have seen cases where a patient is taking a drug for his depression and, while he is experiencing some difficulty maintaining an erection, he can still have sex. However, if a second medication, say for hypertension, is added, his sexual performance will be severely impaired. A complete loss of erectile function can result.

The men in these predicaments have sex lives held hostage by the very medications that can save them. It is an ironic and frustrating situation. I have seen men blame themselves or their partners, not even realizing that their problems had a physiological cause.

Sometimes, men will suspect that the medication mix is responsible for, or contributing to, their hardness problems. On their own, they may decide to try lowered dosages or stop taking the drugs altogether. This very dangerous action can be deadly and must be avoided. In the case of hypertensive medication, lack of the drug may cause blood pressure to suddenly soar to dangerously high levels. The outcome can be a stroke or a heart attack.

Right now, there are more than 200 medications on the market that can seriously compromise erections and sexual performance. Unfortunately, the Food and Drug Administration, the government agency that approves all medications, does not require pharmaceutical companies to reduce potential sexual side effects.

5. HARDNESS FACTOR SOLUTION

When it comes to avoiding certain prescription medications because of their effect on sexual response, there is no simple answer. Not every drug gives the same trouble to each man who uses it. If you suddenly notice that you are having hardness problems where none existed before, take a good look at all medications you are using. Please visit www.thehardnessfactor .com for an extensive listing of medications that can negatively affect hardness.

I recommend that all men 40 and older who have complaints of depression have their testosterone levels checked. This is done with a simple blood test. The reason for this is that if men are found to have suboptimal testosterone levels, testosterone replacement may be a very effective adjunct to their antidepressant medication regimen. The additional testosterone may actually reverse the depression, and after a while antidepressant medications may no longer be needed.

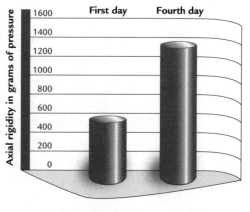

HARDNESS FACTOR
Four-Day Insurance Policy

A 41-year-old male was undergoing testosterone replacement. Baseline readings were adequate for intercourse (**590**), but after following the Four-Day Program he had consistent readings (**912, 976, 1,380**) which represented significant changes in penile axial rigidity. The patient noted that erections seemed to be consistently firmer, and his increased stamina made them easier to sustain.

Patient #P-8 • 41 years old

HARDNESS CHALLENGE SIX:
DIABETES LIMITS ERECTIONS

Type 2 diabetes is a chronic disease most often triggered in adulthood by obesity. The total diabetes rate has tripled over the past thirty years. New federal figures show that 17 million Americans currently have diagnosable Type 2 diabetes and experts estimate that the actual number of at-risk Americans is substantially higher, since obesity, the number-one risk factor for diabetes, remains rampant in children, adolescents, and young adults.

While 5 percent of 30-year-old men have regular hardness problems, approximately 15 percent of men the same age with diabetes have complaints. The problems only worsen with time. Half of the men with diabetes over the age of 50 have erectile problems and getting a sustainable erection is always difficult. That's because the disease damages the tiny nerves responsible for erection. The condition is often made worse by the addition of high blood pressure, obesity, and elevated cholesterol, medical conditions that impact hardness by damaging blood vessels and limiting blood flow.

6. HARDNESS FACTOR SOLUTION

Researchers blame an increasingly sedentary lifestyle and the popular high-fat, high-calorie American fast-food diet for the out-of-control diabetes rates. The large portions that have become a mainstay of the U.S. restaurant industry are also contributing to the diabetes epidemic.

Men can lower their overall diabetes risk by becoming more physically active and losing weight. Unfortunately, even when it is carefully controlled, men with diabetes are still three times more likely to develop erectile dysfunction. Since the disease damages the nerves that trigger erections, prescription erection drugs are often necessary in order to achieve maximum hardness. For those men who have no success with the drugs, special medication injected directly into the penis before lovemaking will induce hardness in minutes. Talk about good news and bad news.

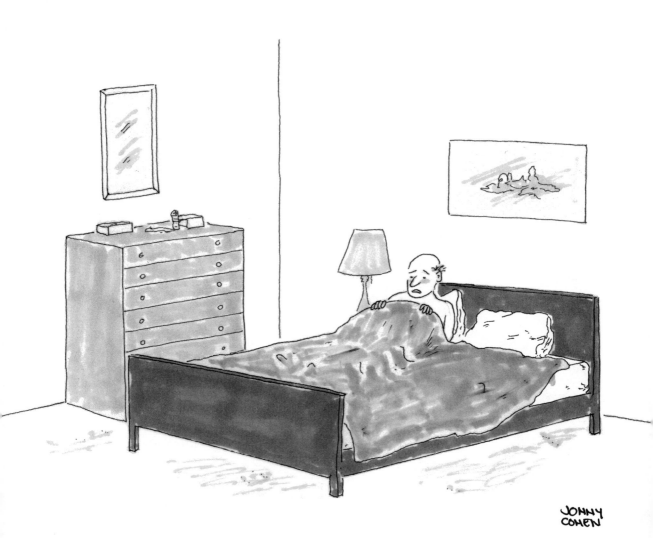

"IS IT ME?"

JONNY
COHEN

66 *Mommy, Mommy. The old man's in the bathroom, and he's got something hard in his pants. . . .*

Curb Your Enthusiasm

12

HARDER PROBLEMS

Millions of men have trouble getting a hard erection on a regular basis. Among them are some of my patients who have tried the Six-Week Program and were unable to significantly enhance their hardness because of underlying medical conditions, which range from diabetes and heart disease, to hypertension and the aftermath of prostate cancer procedures. To these men I say, Thank God for the prescription erection drugs. Remember, however, that an erection is no substitute for the Hardness Factor Program to realize the full potential of these drugs.

THE SUN ALSO SETS

Viagra, the now-legendary blue pill, was approved by the FDA in 1998. Since then, two similar erection-enhancing drugs, Levitra and Cialis, have been approved, offering men a choice.

If these revolutionary erection drugs ultimately change the health habits of men by making them aware that they have an underlying health problem and spurring them to make changes in their lifestyle, they will be considered the most important medications of our generation. However, if the drugs are simply used to improve the hardness of an erection—a Band-Aid to mask symptoms of serious medical problems—only a portion of their potential will be realized. Men need to understand that a hard erection in the absence of improved physical and mental health is not likely to alter their quality of life or result in more sex.

SEXUAL MEDICINE IS MEDICINE

There are some common misconceptions about these hardness drugs. They are not libido enhancers, nor do they cause instant erections after taking them. These drugs will not kill you—unless you happen to take a nitrate-based medication (such as a heart medication containing nitroglycerine) with them. It should also be noted, however, that if your cardiac health status is precarious, the physical activity of sex itself—and not the medication—may contribute to a cardiac event. That said, these highly effective drugs can play a very important role in the restoration of erections for men with chronic mild to severe hardness issues. There is already data that increasingly indicates these drugs are actually good for your heart and blood vessels and will commonly be used in the near future as heart remedies.

Still, some men may find that, try as they might, these erection drugs do not produce a satisfying erection. Granted, some men do have advanced disease that thwarts the effects of the drug, but in many cases, it turns out that the men just don't know how to use the drugs.

Penile Colonies

During religious frenzies in medieval Syria, some Christian men reportedly cut off their own penises and then ran through the towns, eventually tossing their dismembered members on the doorsteps of their fellow townsmen. The households chosen were then obliged to take the young men in and dress them as women. What a drag.

VIAGRA—THE BEGINNING

Researchers have found that many of the men who tried Viagra and said that it didn't work (so-called "Viagra failures") were actually using the drug improperly. Some had taken Viagra after eating a heavy meal, which interferes with the absorption of the medication. Others took a sub-optimal dose (many were taking 50 mg instead of 100 mg, the highest dose), or they expected results too soon after taking the pill. Viagra can take 30 minutes or longer to kick in. Still others completely overlooked the role of sexual stimulation (having the partner more involved in the lovemaking process is important) in providing an erection. Then, too, some men gave up on the drug after trying it just once. Some of the men who had not been having sexual relations for some time were not able to interest their partner in resuming a sex life after the drug restored their erections.

Men need to understand that these drugs are not going to improve a flawed relationship, and that introducing one of these erection medications into a formerly sexless partnership could actually prove to be a powerful destabilizing force. In addition, when your partner's physical and sexual health is impaired, it is going to affect the quality of sex. Therefore, unless your partner's medical issues are addressed, the potential of the drugs will not be realized.

Mistakes such as these may explain in part why many men who have tried Viagra have not renewed their prescriptions. Viagra should be taken on an empty stomach, allowing an hour for it to reach *maximum* strength in the bloodstream. Sexual stimulation will then typically trigger an erection. Many men will find that the drug may work within a half hour or less, but I have found it to be most effective at the one-hour mark.

Try Viagra at least five times and see how you react before deeming it a failure. Actually, before you ever use it for sex with your partner, take it for a "test drive" on your own. Through self-stimulation with the drug on board, you will get comfortable with it and better understand how it works for you and what the possible side effects might be. Once you have built this comfort level, you will be confident in your abilities and ready to involve your partner—but hey, no rush. As Woody Allen remarked in *Annie Hall,* "Hey, don't knock masturbation. It's sex with someone I love."

Guys Need to Know:

- Viagra is an extremely effective agent. The drug that revolutionized the field of sexual medicine is backed by a tremendous amount of clinical research from studies conducted around the world with thousands of men.
- It's effective when used according to doctor's orders: Take on an empty stomach; sexual stimulation is needed.
- Maximum power of the drug is reached in one hour or less.
- Viagra comes in 25 mg, 50 mg, and 100 mg formulations, making it convenient to break the 100 mg pill into two 50 mg pills. I find that 50 mg is extremely effective for the majority of my patients.
- Men with more severe disease will probably need to take 100 mg.
- Viagra may not work if your testosterone levels are too low.
- The drug may cause a stuffy nose and impart a bluish tint to vision when 100 mg dosages are taken.
- Use with caution if also taking alpha-blocking drugs for BPH or hypertension. Alert your physician. Start with the lowest possible dose of ED medication.
- DO NOT USE if taking a nitrate-based medication.

*D*o Not Disturb

A man is in a hotel lobby. He wants to ask the clerk a question. As he turns to go to the front desk, he accidentally bumps into a woman beside him and as he does, his elbow goes into her breast. They are both quite startled. The man turns to her and says, "Ma'am, if your heart is as soft as your breast, I know you'll forgive me." She replies, "If your penis is as hard as your elbow, I'm in room 436."

LEVITRA (2003)

Levitra works as a very potent agent and has been shown in laboratory and clinical trials to be a powerful medication that effectively blocks the erection-deflating action of the enzyme PDE5. This explains why it often works the first time for most men when they try the drug and why 80 percent of the men who have used it have had successful intercourse.

Levitra works within 10 minutes of taking the pill and lasts up to 12 hours. In addition to having a quick onset of action, potency is not adversely affected by being taken with food. The drug is available in 10 mg and 20 mg formulations.

Guys Need to Know:

▶ Levitra is an extremely effective agent. The drug is backed by a tremendous amount of clinical research from studies conducted around the world with thousands of men. Research reported significant improvement in erection hardness and quality.

▶ It's effective when used according to doctor's orders: Sexual stimulation is needed.

▶ Rapid onset of the medication is noted in most men in less than 15 minutes. This is especially a plus for men with psychological problems related to their weak erections—they now have an agent that will work quickly, giving them the confidence to proceed.

▶ Levitra can be taken with food without significant impact on onset of action.

▶ Levitra comes in 10 mg and 20 mg formulations. I find that 10 mg is extremely effective for the majority of my patients.

▶ Men with more severe disease will probably need to take 20 mg.

▶ Levitra may not work if your testosterone levels are too low.

▶ Use with caution if also taking alpha-blocking drugs for BPH or hypertension. Alert your physician. Start with the lowest possible dose of ED medication.

▶ DO NOT USE if taking a nitrate-based medication.

> 66 A significant number of prescription drugs sold online are counterfeit and do not contain the proper dosages.

CIALIS (2003)

Cialis (pronounced See-Alice) is less affected by food consumption and stays in the system for up to 36 hours. The longer duration certainly offers more opportunity for spontaneous lovemaking with no time pressures, which is certainly viewed as a plus by many couples. Take the pill on a Friday night, for example, and you are "good to go" for the weekend—hence the nickame: "Le weekend." Cialis comes in 10 mg and 20 mg dosages, but most men will need the 20 mg dose.

Guys Need to Know:

▶ Cialis is an extremely effective agent. The drug is backed by a tremendous amount of clinical research from studies conducted around the world with thousands of men.

▶ It's effective for up to 36 hours when used according to doctor's orders: Sexual stimulation is needed.

▶ Onset of the medication is noted in many men in less than 30 minutes, but it is best when taken one to two hours before a sexual encounter.

▶ Cialis can be taken with food without significant impact on onset of action.

▶ Many men take advantage of Cialis's multiple-day duration of action so they don't have to plan, rush, or worry about time.

▶ Cialis comes in 5, 10, and 20 mg formulations. I prefer the 20 mg formulation for most of my patients.

▶ Men with severe liver or kidney disease will probably need to take a lower 5 to 10 mg dose due to differences in drug metabolism.

▶ Cialis may not work if your testosterone levels are too low.

▶ Use with caution if also taking alpha-blocking drugs for BPH or hypertension. Alert your physician. Start with the lowest possible dose of ED medication.

▶ DO NOT USE if taking a nitrate-based medication.

ERECTION DRUG SIDE EFFECTS

Cialis, Levitra, and Viagra are well tolerated by most men. Headache, flushing, mild stomach problems, backache (Cialis), and mild visual changes (Viagra) are more of a nuisance than a serious problem for some men and the side effects dissipate the more the drug is used.

Note: Each of these erection drugs can be *lethal* if taken at the same time with any nitrate-based medication and in those men with significant underlying heart disease that prevents them from undertaking physical exertion.

WHICH ERECTION DRUG TO CHOOSE

What has become very clear to me is that each of the erection drugs is very effective. When it comes to choosing an erection drug, I tell my patients to try all three and then see which works best for them and suits their particular needs. While men come to develop favorites, a recent international study of the three drugs found that one-third of the men preferred Viagra, one-third liked Levitra, and one-third found Cialis to be their favorite. Every man has a distinct perception of what sex is and what feels the most natural with his penis and his partner.

Each drug works very well for mild to moderate ED. More severe dysfunction will require a higher dose of a particular drug. Great erections should not be confused with great sexual relationships. Ultimately, the real success of these drugs depends on sexual intimacy and a strong relationship with your partner.

BUYING ERECTION DRUGS ON THE INTERNET

In the marketplace, it is always caveat emptor—buyer beware—and it's no different when buying anything on the Internet, where there are more than 1,400 pharmacy sites. Studies have reported that a significant number of prescription drugs sold online are counterfeit and do not contain the proper dosages, or any of the actual ingredients of the purported medication being sold. Many of these unscrupulous websites work out of third-world countries and are far from the reach of the FDA and most law enforcement agencies from other countries.

OTHER ERECTILE DYSFUNCTION TREATMENT OPTIONS

When advanced erectile dysfunction causes even the three oral medications to fail, it is time to contact a urologist. Urologists are medical experts who specialize in the prevention and treatment of male urological problems, which include sexual health medication issues. And just as women seek the help of gynecological specialists for their sexual health medication problems, men need to avail themselves of expert urological advice when it comes to advanced hardness problems. When the erection drugs no longer work, there are several hardness options to consider with your urologist. Let's review each of them:

Penile Injection. A very effective therapy, even for men with ED caused by prostate surgery. Special erection-inducing drugs are injected into the side of the penis 5 to 20 minutes before sexual intercourse.

Vacuum Erection Device. Very effective therapy for all types of ED. Simply place the penis in the plastic tube and pump the device to create an erection.

Penile Implant Surgery. The most effective therapy for men with advanced ED. Produces hard erections instantly for everyone.

ERECTILE DYSFUNCTION THERAPY

THERAPY	EFFECTIVENESS	DIRECTIONS
Viagra	Very effective for up to 4–5 hours when used according to instructions. Less effective for men with diabetes and will not work with men who have had both erection nerves removed during prostate cancer surgery.	Best when taken 1 hour before a sexual encounter, but may take 15–30 minutes to work. Less effective if taken with food. Available in 25 mg, 50 mg, and 100 mg formulations. 50 mg is a common starting dose; some may need 100 mg. Do not take more than one pill in a 24-hour span.
Levitra	Very effective for up to 10–12 hours when used according to instructions. Very potent. No visual effects. Less effective for men with diabetes and will not work with men who have had both erection nerves removed during prostate cancer surgery.	Best when taken 30–60 minutes prior to a sexual encounter, but can be highly effective in as little as 10 minutes. Less affected by food. Available in 10 mg and 20 mg formulations. Do not take more than one pill in a 24-hour span.
Cialis	Very effective for up to 36 hours when used according to instructions. Very potent. No visual effects. Less effective for men with diabetes and will not work with men who have had both erection nerves removed during prostate cancer surgery.	Best when taken 1 hour before a sexual encounter, but can be highly effective in 30 minutes. Less affected by food. Available in 10 mg and 20 mg formulations. Do not take more than one pill in a 24-hour span.

> ❝ *It's as satisfying to me as, uh, coming is, you know? As, ah, having sex with a woman and coming. And so can you believe how much I am in heaven? I am like, uh, getting the feeling of coming in a gym, I'm getting the feeling of coming at home, I'm getting the feeling of coming backstage when I pump up, when I pose in front of 5,000 people, I get the same feeling, so I am coming day and night. I mean, it's terrific. Right? So you know, I am in heaven.*

Arnold Schwarzenegger,
Pumping Iron

13

HARDER STILL

After having followed the Six-Week Program (or at least having read this far) and realizing how your health and hardness are so intertwined, I want you to know that the program offers even more. The recent discovery about the impact of nitric oxide on cardiac and penile function, as well as the evolution of functional fitness in this country, now means that following this program will not only improve your libido and hardness, but as you continue to follow the program daily, it will help enhance muscle definition, slim and trim your physique, and allow you to enjoy life, looking and feeling great.

ENOUGH ABOUT THE PENIS

Hardness, of course, is not just about the quality of one's erection. Performing functional exercises using your own body weight as resistance does more to ensure overall physical well-being than just about anything I know. Muscle is the most metabolically active tissue you have in your body. Think of your muscles as a huge furnace that is always switched on. Strengthening your muscles daily with the assortment of simple upper- and lower-body exercises in my sexual fitness routine are already helping to stoke that internal furnace, paring off excess fat and replacing it with muscle. For every pound of muscle you put on, expect to burn an additional 100 calories per day. This helps reverse the slow but steady weight gain among Americans that impacts both health and hardness.

By the way, the special L-arginine and Pycnogenol mixture you have been taking since the first week to enhance nitric oxide (NO) production in your penis is also helping add to your overall muscle-building capabilities. The extra NO helps dilate blood vessels, which means more blood can get to your muscles when you exercise them. When your muscles become engorged with blood, the muscle's outer sheath is stretched, helping the muscle to grow in size. As you begin to get in shape, you are going to look and feel better.

Fear of Ugliness

MARK, age 26—I'm so pretty

Mark was a new patient and he had some hardness concerns, most likely linked to his erratic sleep patterns. But he came to me not to talk about his erections but to get clearance for an upcoming surgical procedure.

Rugged and powerfully built, the 26-year-old Mark mentioned that he had always been upset by the size of his calf muscles. "They are too scrawny," he said matter-of-factly as he sat in my examination room. But he told me that he had finally found a way to deal with the undersized muscles. In three weeks, he was going to a plastic surgeon to have silicone implants put into his calves to bulk them up.

I was taken aback. Mark's calf muscles seemed perfectly proportioned. Still, Mark said he had always been too embarrassed to wear shorts or go to the beach. "I know people are staring at my calves because they are so emaciated. I lift weights all the time, but it doesn't help. I feel like a freak. And I'm curious, Dr. Lamm, who would you recommend for penis enhancement? I read that they can take fat from other parts of your body and inject it into the penis to make it bigger. I find that I am on the small size compared to other men."

While taking Mark's medical history, I realized that the upcoming calf-implant surgery would not be his first foray into the world of cosmetic plastic surgery procedures. Four years earlier, he had his nose reshaped. "It was just too crooked," he explained. The following year, it was his ears. "Everyone would always stare at me," he said. "I drove my girlfriend crazy because I would always talk about how hideous they were. Shortly after we broke up, I found another plastic surgeon and had my ears pinned back. The doctor did an okay job, but not great."

Mark's nose and ears looked perfectly normal. His penis, like his calf muscles, was also normal. It was becoming clear to me that this handsome man with well-proportioned features actually hated the way he looked. I told Mark that I was concerned about him. Since he already had multiple plastic surgeries, I explained that he might be suffering from what is known as body dysmorphic disorder (BDD), a poorly understood psychiatric disorder that is closely related to obsessive-compulsive disorder.

People with BDD—and it is estimated that it affects as many as 5 million American men and women—become so preoccupied with their imagined or real physical flaws that it leads to a compulsive checking and rechecking in mirrors throughout the day, as well as inappropriate surgeries.

The tip-off to me that a person has BDD is that the degree of deformity perceived by the patient is much greater than that which should be observed by a normal person. The hair on the back of my neck stands up whenever a person asks for a procedure that doesn't seem in the realm of reality. Many physical problems can be

*T*he Grecian Formula

Male nudity in ancient Greece, particularly among young athletes, was common. A forerunner of the modern jockstrap, the kynodesme or dog knot, was employed. A man would cover the head of his penis with the foreskin and tie it with a leather strip. He would then knot the two ends of the strip to the base of his penis.

*L*ittle Big Man

In ancient Greece, a small penis was considered the ideal.

fixed through surgery. However, for people with BDD, the problem is psychiatric, not physical, and many of these people will never be satisfied with the results of any plastic surgery.

I did not clear Mark for the implant surgery and suggested instead that he make an appointment with one of my psychiatric colleagues for treatment. BDD treatment that combines the use of cognitive (talk) therapy and a daily drug regimen can be very effective in helping people deal with their distorted body image and compulsive behavior. Unfortunately, Mark did not follow up with my colleague and I never saw him again. It was disturbing.

SURFACE LESSONS

Lesson 1   A concern about your physical appearance is healthy and contributes to your overall self-confidence.

Lesson 2   Size is a matter of perception, not pleasure or virility.

Lesson 3   Obsessing excessively about a particular body part that is considered unattractive—body dysmorphic disorder (BDD)—is cause for concern.

Lesson 4   BDD, or "imagined ugliness," can affect work, social, and personal functioning.

Lesson 5   BDD should be treated by a mental health professional.

MY HARDNESS WORKOUT

The exercise component of the Hardness Factor Program is the one variable that is totally under your control. Look at the Six-Week Program I have detailed in the previous chapters as the basic map that puts you on the road to hardness. I have set the minimum requirements. Some of you may already exercise more than I recommend in the Six-Week Program, and that is certainly fantastic. Some of you will read on and find that you already far exceed what I do each week, which is even better.

The bottom line with exercise: The more one does, the greater the benefit for heart, hardness, and health. Stay motivated to run, walk, swim, bike, hike, kayak, or lift weights throughout the year by focusing simply on the pleasure you derive from it.

Two decades ago, my training mainly consisted of jogging so I could be in shape to play tennis. With more research coming out that pointed to the benefits of strength training, I began lifting weights several times a week for power and endurance. Functional Fitness, which incorporated a variety of exercises that helped make me more limber and strong in performing the motions of everyday activities, really caught my attention about four years ago.

On Monday, Wednesday, and Friday I end my workday by heading off to a local gym to exercise. Twice a week I perform functional exercises with weights and my own body weight, while the third session is devoted to lifting weights. I warm up with a run on the treadmill and make the ten minutes count by constantly pushing myself with an interval workout—spurts of intense exertion alternating with lower-intensity recovery periods.

I start running at 6 mph (10-minute mile) and at the three-minute mark, I sprint for thirty seconds with the treadmill moving at a 6.5 mph pace. Dropping back to 6 mph for a minute, I then sprint for another thirty seconds with the treadmill moving at 7 mph. If Suzie, my extremely fit daughter, happens to be working out with me, the pace is even faster.

I have to challenge myself every day and I push myself to meet my changing goals. My interval training, which consists of multiple thirty-second bursts of sprinting interspersed with running slower for one minute, gets my heart pounding, oftentimes approaching 150 beats per minute, almost tripling my resting heart rate.

Warm-up done, I am now ready for some challenging functional exercises. You can only get harder if you make your workouts harder, so the repetitions for these special exercises I have performed for the past two weeks will go up by three for each exercise starting today.

Of all the resistance exercises, I like bench pressing the most. The steady rhythm and muscle pump mentally and physically prepare me for what lies ahead for the next half hour. My upper back flat on the oversized red Swiss ball, I quickly knock out a set of 12 repetitions with the barbell. The trick with this exercise comes in maintaining balance through the abdomen as you push the weights up and down.

Taking some weight off the bar, I go through a set of biceps curls. What adds functionality to this exercise is that I do it while standing balanced atop a BOSU, a device that looks like a small stability ball cut in half. My abdominal muscles contract fully as I curl the bar up to my shoulders. By the tenth repetition, my arms are on fire as I struggle to stay on the BOSU.

The gym starts to fill up with other people coming in after work, but I hardly notice. I am focused, and in "the zone." Grabbing a pair of dumbbells, I get back on the BOSU and go through a series of dumbbell overhead shoulder presses, one arm up and over my head at a time. My arms and abdominal muscles are quivering as I strain to stay on the BOSU and complete my reps.

Next come squats. Holding the weights at my sides, I attempt to lower myself into a squat position until my thighs are almost horizontal. My legs are burning and sweat is pouring onto the floor by the last repetition. This exercise is very important because, in addition to building the muscles of my thighs and buttocks, it delivers huge quantities of blood to my pelvic area.

I finish with some calf raises that leave my lower legs drained from the exertion and then head back to the bench press, ready to repeat the same series of exercises again. The second round of exercises is even harder to complete, but I push myself to finish.

"Pulled it off," I say to myself as I towel off and head for the showers, happy in the rush of another post-workout high. I've performed more repetitions than the week before, but better yet, I feel revitalized, more energetic than I did a mere thirty minutes earlier. It's amazing how exercise, actually an adult form of "play time," can make you feel so alive.

I call my wife. Dinner. Dancing. Romancing. There's not a better way to end a busy day.

Sweat Equity

DAVID, age 32—Lifting down the numbers

The blood work came back and David was not happy. At 32, the hard-driving consultant had a cholesterol level of 255 mg/dL. In lieu of starting him on a lifetime of statin medication to keep his cholesterol in check, I gave him an option. "Start a regular functional training program, working out three times a week for the next eight weeks," I told him. "If you are able to drop your LDL cholesterol and build up your HDL levels, and agree to continue with the weight training program, then I will not start you on the medication." David readily agreed and we went over some training exercises I thought he might enjoy.

David's next cholesterol test was much better, with an HDL level now at 48, a five-point boost. He also dropped 30 points on his LDL level. Eliminating body fat, building muscle, and cutting back on the fatty foods that made up a good part of his diet all played important roles in David's new cholesterol profile. I told him that if he was able to keep up this new regimen, I was convinced that he would eventually get his cholesterol into the safe range.

> ## SWEATY LESSONS
>
> **Lesson 1**   You can make significant alterations in your lipid profile through relatively simple lifestyle changes.
>
> **Lesson 2**   A lifetime of prescription medication will be required to lower your heart risks (and maintain some level of hardness) if you cannot or will not make appropriate lifestyle modifications.

WHY WEIGHT?

Resistance training, whether it is with your own body weight, iron plates, or weight-training machines, builds lean body tissue—that's muscle—and cranks up your metabolism. When the process by which the body converts the calories in food to energy is speeded up, you can make steady and significant gains in how you look and feel, beginning with the very first resistance workout. Keep training on a regular basis (I like to work out at least three times a week), and you can:

Get a testosterone (libido) boost. Regular resistance training increases levels of testosterone, the powerful male sex hormone. The more muscle you have and the leaner you are, the more testosterone you will have circulating in your blood.

Enhance sexual pleasure. Sex is a whole-body experience, so it makes sense that you'll enjoy it more when your heart, muscles, and blood vessels are performing at peak levels, thanks to having muscles that are more powerful.

Pare off pounds of excess body fat. As you increase muscle strength and hardness, your body will become leaner and you will have more stamina.

Speed up metabolism. Muscles are the most metabolically active tissues of the body. Think of them as engines that are always turned on. For every pound of muscle you put on, expect to burn an additional 100 calories per day. Even when your muscles are at rest, and this includes when you are sleeping, your muscles keep burning calories.

Improve the functioning of your heart. Like your other muscles, the heart becomes stronger and larger because of weight training. A fit heart will pump more blood at this maximum level and can sustain it longer with less strain.

Combat excess blood sugar. Resistance training builds muscle, increasing the sensitivity of cells to insulin, which, in turn, lowers blood sugar and the need for insulin. This helps prevent adult-onset diabetes.

Boost your "good" cholesterol level. Cholesterol, a waxy substance found in the bloodstream, helps form cell membranes, some hormones, and a variety of tissues. Lifting weights on a regular basis boosts protective HDL (the "good" cholesterol) levels, while lowering LDL ("bad" cholesterol) blood levels. The higher your HDL level (the ideal is defined as 60 mg/dL or more), the more protection you have against coronary artery disease.

Enable your body to move more efficiently. The exercises strengthen what tends to get weak and stretch what tends to get tight.

Boost self-confidence. Regular training can enhance overall feelings of well-being, making you feel both confident and attractive. Sexual Fitness doesn't replace resistance or functional training workouts, and vice versa. The secret is to both challenge your muscles and integrate them for total support and strength.

NO: GOOD FOR THE PUMP

Arnold Schwarzenegger, the former Mr. Olympia bodybuilding champion and now the governor of California, once mentioned to a startled audience on *The Oprah Winfrey Show* that when he trains in the gym with weights, the "pump is better than coming."

While many might disagree somewhat with the comparison between weight training effects and orgasm, for the millions of men who have trained with weights, they know exactly what Arnold means.

By the third and final set of lifting or pushing a heavy weight in the gym, it often becomes a mighty struggle as you summon all of your muscles—as well as your psychological staying power—to make it through to the tenth and final rep. When the weight is finally down, however, you get the big payoff. You feel *pumped.*

You're pumped because you have triggered the release of nitric oxide in the body. This special molecule helps dilate your blood vessels, allowing more oxygen- and nutrient-rich blood to pour in, nourishing and enlarging your fatigued muscles in the process.

And yes, it does feel great when the muscles are pumped. It's a good feeling when you have finished the final set. It is also good to know that your muscles are growing and that you are getting harder and stronger. Is the pump as good as an orgasm? Well, that's for you to decide.

Nitric oxide is a truly remarkable vascular agent that scientists are still trying to understand. Researchers are now harnessing it and using it in novel medical therapies with newborns to make it easier for them to breathe. NO is also being used to

It Only Comes in Hardcover

Norwegian sexologists published a "Penis Atlas" in 2004, in which one hundred men's penises were photographed, to clarify and correct many misunderstandings about the male sex organ.

help people overcome the life-threatening blood vessel disorder known as pulmonary hypertension, as well as to help prevent the formation of lethal blood clots in the body.

While scientists are still discovering new and varied uses for NO, I want to remind you that the sexual exercise program you perform each week also triggers the release of hundreds of thousands of NO molecules, allowing for maximum expansion of the internal diameter of your penile blood vessels. The result is maximum hardness. Is orgasm as good as the pump? Again, that's for you to decide.

Now that the six weeks of the program are over, I want you to give serious thought to taking your hardness efforts to the next level. This means moving from the body weight exercises that I outlined for you to more demanding barbell or dumbbell sessions using a Swiss ball or BOSU board, or traditional weight-machine workouts. You have much to gain.

It wasn't that long ago that exercise experts thought that weight training was for narcissistic bodybuilders who spent hours every day hoisting weights and staring at themselves in floor-to-ceiling mirrors. Actually, as the scientists found out, there was more to weight training than mere vanity. Much more in fact. Take your hardness workouts to the next level. And why not? Hard is good, but harder is even better.

IT'S YOUR BODY, HOW HARD DO YOU WANT IT?

By now you have discovered the awesome power that a variety of small changes can make in the physical, psychological, and emotional elements that make up a fulfilling sex life. You've also seen how knowledge about the workings of the penis, daily exercise and stretching sessions, different supplements, and sensual eating can make a big difference in your hardness and overall enjoyment of sex. The past six weeks have been a journey of self-discovery and I am privileged to have been your guide.

But the rest is all up to you. How you succeed, how you get over the many hurdles thrown in your path every day all comes down to you. How much do you really want to get harder? How much do you really want to become healthier? I have shown you how to live better. It's up to you to accept the responsibility to live that life. It's difficult.

Although the book ends here, I want you to start thinking about Week Seven and how you can successfully work all of the changes into your lifestyle and move forward to Weeks Eight, Nine, Ten, and beyond. To increase and maintain your hardness, you will have to continue to incorporate all the many concepts from the previous weeks. As you progress, notice how much more energy you have. How much stronger you feel. How much harder you have become.

> 66 You are now an active and healthy man. You are a hard man.

Perhaps, though, you might feel a little overwhelmed. The changes you have to make are so many that you don't know what to do. If that sounds like you, then I encourage you to go back and reread the material for each week of the program so you fully understand what is expected of you. Repeat the entire program. You will only become harder as you adopt the many lifestyle changes.

It's never too late and you're never too old to begin the Hardness Factor Program. You want to maximize your health, don't you? Then begin today. Start eliminating those bad health habits. Don't delay. Put health and hardness first in your life.

For those of you who have successfully integrated the principles of the Hardness Factor into your life, I congratulate you. You stepped back and reviewed your health and hardness during the first week of the program. You took positive measures to enhance and preserve it over the weeks to the best of your ability. In doing so, you created a new image for yourself. You are now an active and healthy man. You are a hard man.

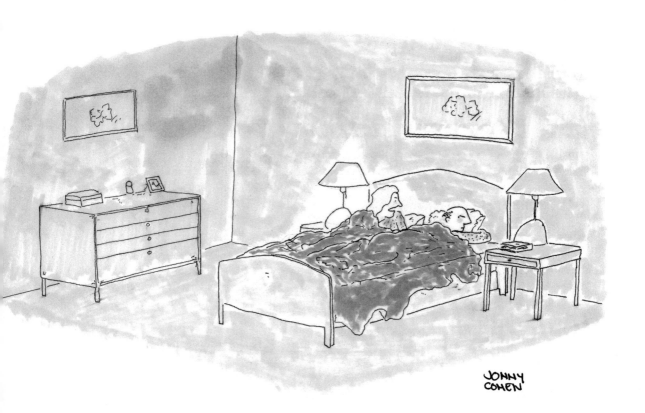

"SOMETIMES, YES MEANS YES."

66 *I've just returned from America, a country of many prominent erections.*

Edward Pierce,
The First Great Train Robbery

APPENDICES

66 *If it's still squishy like the raw breast, it isn't done. And if it's hard, it is, uh, it's overdone, which is too bad.*

Julia Child,
The French Chef Cookbook

Appendix I

EATING HARD

SPECIAL NOTE:
Additional information about the Hardness Factor Program, including tips, exercises, and an assortment of products can be found at www.thehardnessfactor.com

CREATING A HARDNESS-FRIENDLY SHOPPING LIST

I want you to try to shop for food regularly. Veer away from prepared, frozen, canned, and packaged foodstuffs. The more natural the product, the better it is for you. Try to find out where your food comes from. Use organic, local products whenever available. "Support your local farmers market," says Waldy. "They typically offer the best quality and price for the freshest foods around."

Also, be sure to avoid trans-fatty acids, or trans fats, which are often found in commercial baked goods, snack foods, and stick margarine. Some experts believe they are as bad as animal fats in raising cholesterol levels and increasing the risk of heart disease. However, according to the rules of the Food and Drug Administration, trans fat content does not have to appear on food labels. Therefore, be on the lookout for foods labeled "hydrogenated" on the list of ingredients. Margarines, snacks, and prepared foods have oils that have been hydrogenated into trans fats to keep them solid at room temperature, thereby increasing shelf life.

To boost your energy levels, health, and hardness, you need to create a hardness-friendly shopping list. Here are the basic foods Waldy Malouf suggests you incorporate into your hardness diet:

1. Apples. In ancient times, the Swedes believed apples were the food of the gods, while Greeks and Romans threw them to lovers as a means of enticement. In modern times, an apple a day actually can keep the doctor away with its insoluble and soluble fiber (including pectin), some vitamin C, and potassium. Apples are also an excellent source of quercetin, a flavonoid known to protect against heart disease.

2. Arugula. This leafy vegetable, a member of the broccoli family, supplies folic acid and some calcium and contains cancer-fighting phytochemicals called indoles. Arugula's dark green color and pungent flavor are an indication that it also contains some beta-carotene and vitamin C. Known also as "rocket" salad, arugula historically has been known to boost sagging libidos.

3. Asparagus. This purported aphrodisiac—because of its phallic shape—contains the phytochemical glutathione, which has excellent antioxidant properties. Asparagus also has a good supply of folic acid and some vitamin C.

4. Avocado. This fruit, reminiscent of a woman's body, seems almost too delicious to be healthful. However, avocados contain a significant amount of a cholesterol-lowering molecule called beta-sitosterol. The fat in avocados is monounsaturated, the type that benefits a hard penis and healthy heart. Avocados are rich in vitamin E, another antioxidant hardness helper. This vegetable with a velvety mouth feel provides substantial amounts of folic acid, vitamin B_6, and some iron and magnesium.

5. Banana. Nearly an ideal food, bananas have much to offer nutritionally. This phallic-shaped fruit supplies a substantial amount of potassium along with significant amounts of vitamin B_6. Bananas also have a small amount of vitamin C and folic acid.

6. Blueberries. As a snack or dessert, this is the one food that is highest in disease-fighting antioxidants. Anthocyanins, a group of substances that put the "blue" in the fruit, are responsible for much of the antioxidant power of the berry. In addition, blueberries have a high fiber content, with much of that fiber in the form of pectin, a soluble fiber that helps lower cholesterol levels.

7. Carrots. The ancient Romans thought sexual hardness was directly linked to what a person ate. The shape, color, and flavor of food determined its impact on one's sex life. Therefore, root vegetables such as carrots became instant symbols of strength of libido. Vitamin A is derived from beta-carotene and carrots are a major source of this substance. This ever-popular phallic-like vegetable is also a source of disease-fighting flavonoids, which contain calcium pectate, a type of fiber that is thought to help reduce blood cholesterol levels.

8. Chili peppers. It's their mouth-watering flavor (some refer to it as a "burn") that attracts the most attention, but chili peppers are also packed with vitamin C, the antioxidant powerhouse that helps fight free radicals in the body. Capsaicin, the compound that provides the hot spice and heat, helps lower LDL cholesterol and thins the blood as well. Eating these tiny fire pellets causes the body to become heated, the pulse to quicken, and the face to become flushed—as in a lovemaking session—and triggers the release of endorphins, brain substances that erase the sensation of pain and replace it with pleasure.

9. Chocolate. A genuine "love food," this delicious sweet contains phenylethylamine, the same pleasure-producing chemical released when we fall in love. Chocolate is good for your heart and hardness, containing hundreds of chemicals with benefits ranging from cardiovascular protection to immune defense. Catechin, the same flavonoid found in tea, is abundant in chocolate, and it is thought to help reduce LDL cholesterol levels in the blood.

10. Cucumbers. Cukes, a good source of fiber, are crisp, cool, and moist because of their high water content. Their sexually stimulating qualities are linked to their phallic appearance.

11. Fennel. These tiny flavor-packed yellow-brown seeds are thought to stimulate sexual desire.

12. Figs. Symbolic of the male and female sex organs, sweet figs are a superb source of fiber, potassium, iron, and calcium.

13. Garlic. Garlic is one of the most potent disease fighters in the plant world. Most of the health benefits derive from the more than one hundred sulfur compounds it contains, especially allicin, which is responsible for its characteristic scent and flavor. Garlic can slow the buildup of plaque on the arteries, prevent the formation of blood clots, and help lower blood pressure, all of which leads to stronger erections. Just be careful of your allicin-scented breath.

14. Ginger. The ginger root looks like some crude phallic symbol, but this spice is one of the most popular in the world because of its pungent taste. Its medicinal value is prized, too, for ginger can help relax blood vessels and boost blood flow.

15. Grapes. An excellent dessert or snack, this fruit is a source of vitamin C.

16. Honey. This "nectar of Aphrodite" has its roots firmly in history, going all the way back to ancient cave paintings. Not only does honey add flavor to numerous foods, but it is a natural sweetener that contains small amounts of amino acids and pinocembrin, an important compound with antioxidant-like activity.

17. Nuts. Recent research found that consuming 5 ounces of nuts a week can cut heart attack likelihood by one-third. Nuts are rich in arginine, the amino acid that helps keep coronary arteries open and clear. Although nuts are high in fat, it is the good kind: monounsaturated and/or omega-3. In addition, nuts supply a variety of minerals, including magnesium, copper, and zinc.

18. Olive oil, extra-virgin. This is the tasty oil that is made from the first pressing of the green olives. Olive oil is the main dietary reason for the decreased risk of heart disease in men living in Mediterranean countries. Compared to the saturated fats typically found in butter, dairy, and meat, the "good" (monounsaturated) fats in extra-virgin olive oil help decrease free radical damage in the coronary arteries, slashing the risk of developing athero-sclerosis. "Whenever possible," says Waldy, "use extra-virgin olive oil in your meal preparation. In addition to raising the level of HDL cholesterol, the olive oil contains a healthy mix of flavonoids and antioxidants."

19. Salmon. One of the most delicious fish, this fatty species contains high amounts of the type of fat—omega-3—that performs miracles throughout the body, the heart especially. It does so by lowering triglyceride levels and blood pressure.

20. Spinach. It is not going to give you the muscle power of Popeye, but it is going to help you nonetheless. Rich in carotenoids, including beta-carotene and lutein, fresh spinach also contains levels of quercetin, a phytochemical with antioxidant properties. Spinach is rich in vitamins and minerals, particularly vitamin K, magnesium, and manganese. In addition, it has plenty of folic acid, which helps prevent heart disease and cancer. Avoid cooking spinach too long; this reduces its nutritional content.

21. Tea. Tea leaves contain potent antioxidant chemicals called polyphenols that help guard against many kinds of basic cell damage. One cup of green or black tea per day cuts heart disease risk in half. Buy it loose or in tea bags.

22. Tomatoes. This ancient aphrodisiac, known as "pomme d'amour," or "love apple," in France, is a great source of vitamins C and A. The red pigment of the tomato is the source of the powerful antioxidant lycopene, which has

Code Orange

A guy goes to a doctor and says, "Doc, you've got to help me. My penis is orange."

The doctor asks the man to drop his pants so he can check. Sure enough, the man's penis is orange. The doctor says to the guy, "This is very strange. Sometimes things like this are caused by a lot of stress in a person's life." Probing as to the causes of possible stress, the doctor asks the man, "How are things going at work?"

The man explains that he was fired about six weeks ago. The doctor tells him that this must be the cause of the stress. The man says, "No. My boss was a real jerk, I had to work 20–30 hours of overtime every week, and I had no say in anything that was happening. I found a new job a couple of weeks ago where I can set my own hours. I'm getting paid double what I got on the old job, and my new boss is a really great guy."

So, the doctor decides this probably wasn't the reason. He asks the guy, "How's your home life?" The guy says, "Well, I got divorced about eight months ago."

The doctor figures that this has got to be the reason for all of the man's stress. But the man says, "No. For years, all I listened to was nag, nag, nag. Jeez, am I glad to be rid of her!"

Baffled, the doctor finally asks, "Do you have any hobbies or a social life?"

The man says, "No, not really. Most nights I just sit at home, watch some porno flicks, and munch on Cheetos."

been shown to prevent the buildup of cholesterol on artery walls. One European study of more than 1,000 men reported that those who consumed the most lycopene in their diets had their risk of heart attack cut in half. Scientists also believe that this important carotenoid may also boost the sperm count of men with depressed levels of lycopene.

23. Whole grains. Grains are hard to beat for their nutritional wallop. They are a prime source of the complex carbohydrates that help to sustain energy. Whole grains contain anticancer agents and help stabilize blood sugar and insulin levels, which are vital for health, fitness, and hardness.

Appendix II

RECIPES FOR HARDNESS

EATING IS A GOOD THING—
SO IS BEING HARD

When I first met Dr. Lamm at the Beacon Restaurant & Bar in New York, where I am the chef and co-owner, I was immediately struck by his notion of sensual cooking, first as a way to lure more men into the kitchen, and second, as a way to teach them to prepare meals that both invigorate the palate and set the table for romance.

More important, however, was Dr. Lamm's desire to come up with great examples of how creative and healthy a man can be when he prepares and consumes a daily diet that not only aids in the prevention of cardiovascular disease but also preserves and maintains sexual performance.

Many people describe eating as an orgasmic experience. I happen to agree. Eating and sex involve virtually the same senses: Smell. Sight. Touch. The idea behind the following fifteen recipes isn't just to prepare two of these dinners each week. Rather, think of these meals as an important starting point, a powerful and delicious way to help change your way of thinking about eating and hardness all life long.

—Waldy Malouf

WEEK ONE

MENU ONE (see page 84)

HERB-CRUSTED SALMON WITH HORSERADISH BREAD SAUCE

Chilled Yellow Tomato Soup
Herb-Crusted Salmon with
Horseradish Bread Sauce
Chocolate Angel Food Cake with
Brandied Strawberries

CHILLED YELLOW TOMATO SOUP

Difficulty: Medium
Prep Time: 30 minutes
Cook Time: 1 hour
Servings: 6

Waldy Says: Make this soup a day ahead. The tomatoes, peppers, herbs, and spices will excite all your senses. The best tasting antioxidant you will ever have.

FOR THE SOUP:
6 large yellow tomatoes
2½ tablespoons extra-virgin olive oil
1 teaspoon coarse sea salt or kosher salt,
    plus additional to taste
1 cup chopped onion
2 garlic cloves, minced
1 teaspoon whole coriander seed
½ teaspoon whole cumin seed
1½ cups water
1 tablespoon fresh lemon juice
½ teaspoon freshly ground black pepper

FOR THE CILANTRO-ONION RELISH:
1 medium red tomato, seeded and diced
½ cup finely chopped red onion
¼ cup chopped cilantro

1 tablespoon fresh lime juice
1 tablespoon extra-virgin olive oil
1 teaspoon minced jalapeno
Coarse sea salt or kosher salt to taste
Freshly ground black pepper to taste

1. Light the grill or preheat the oven to 500°F. Place the tomatoes in a bowl and toss them with 1½ tablespoons olive oil and salt to taste.

2. On the grill: Place the whole tomatoes on the grill for 10 to 15 minutes, turning until the tomatoes are charred. In the oven: Place the whole tomatoes in a roasting pan and roast for 10 minutes. Turn the tomatoes over and roast for another 5 minutes.

3. Transfer the tomatoes to a bowl and let cool slightly. Core and roughly chop them, reserving their juices. Heat the remaining tablespoon of oil in a large pot over medium heat. Add the onions and garlic and cook, stirring, until they are translucent, about 5 minutes. Do not let them brown (if they start to color, add a tablespoon of water).

4. Meanwhile, in a small skillet, toast the coriander and cumin over medium-high heat until they are fragrant and lightly browned, shaking the pan so the spices don't burn, about 2 minutes. Add them to the pot, along with the tomatoes and their liquid, and water. Stir in 1 teaspoon salt.

5. Bring the tomato mixture to a boil over high heat, then reduce the heat and simmer for about 15 minutes.

6. Turn off the heat and let the soup cool slightly. Purée the soup either with an immersion blender, or in batches in a blender or food processor. Strain through a coarse sieve and discard the solids. Chill the soup until cold, at least 4 hours.

7. Season soup with lemon juice, salt to taste, and pepper.

8. Meanwhile, in a bowl, stir together all the ingredients for the cilantro-onion relish.

9. Serve soup garnished with a spoonful of the cilantro-onion relish.

HERB-CRUSTED SALMON WITH HORSERADISH BREAD SAUCE

Difficulty: Medium
Prep Time: 30 minutes
Cook Time: 15 minutes
Servings: 4

Waldy Says: This is a very old-fashioned sauce based on the idea of using stale bread as an emulsifying agent to make what is essentially an egg-less mayonnaise. Here I add pungent horseradish, which is a natural with salmon, and plenty of herbs. Then I garnish the plate with a drizzle of herb oil for a colorful contrast.

½ cup chopped, fresh flat leaf parsley
¼ cup chopped fresh dill, plus additional sprigs
    for garnish
1 tablespoon chopped fresh tarragon
1 small shallot, minced
3 tablespoons freshly squeezed lemon juice,
    or to taste
¼ cup plus 1 tablespoon prepared horseradish
Coarse sea salt or kosher salt to taste
Freshly ground black pepper to taste
⅓ cup plus 3 tablespoons extra-virgin olive oil
4 skinless salmon fillets (1½ inches thick)
½ cup fresh breadcrumbs

1. In the bowl of a food processor or blender, combine the parsley, dill, tarragon, shallot, 1 tablespoon lemon juice, 1 tablespoon horseradish, and a large pinch each salt and pepper. With the motor running, drizzle in 3 tablespoons olive oil, to form a thin paste. Reserve ¼ cup of this herb paste to use for garnish.

2. Lay the salmon in a pan in a single layer and brush with the remaining herb paste, turning to coat both sides of the fish. Cover and refrigerate for at least 20 minutes and up to 2 hours.

3. Preheat the oven to 500°F. Unwrap the salmon.

4. Place the salmon in a roasting pan and roast until done to taste, about 9 to 12 minutes.

5. While the salmon is cooking, place the breadcrumbs in the bowl of a food processor or blender with the remaining ¼ cup horseradish, 1 tablespoon lemon juice, and a pinch of salt and pepper. Blend to combine. With the motor running, drizzle in the remaining ⅓ cup of olive oil, and process until bread sauce is smooth.

6. Whisk the remaining tablespoon of lemon juice into the reserved herb paste, adding a little more olive oil if necessary, so that it becomes a pourable herb oil.

7. To serve, place a pool of the bread sauce on each plate, top with a salmon fillet, and then drizzle the fish and plate with the herb oil and garnish with fresh dill sprigs.

CHOCOLATE ANGEL FOOD CAKE WITH BRANDIED STRAWBERRIES

Difficulty: Medium
Prep Time: 30 minutes
Cook Time: 1 hour 15 minutes
Servings: 8 to 10

Waldy Says: I consider this angel's food, but maybe for angels with a dark side. I make this version even better by serving toasted slices of cake with strawberries that have been roasted until their juices are syrupy and almost caramelized. I find that all red berries work well here, their fresh fruitiness and concentrated sauce complementing the chocolate for a relatively light, summery dessert. The flavonoids in the chocolate and the vitamins in the berries will excite you mentally and physically.

FOR THE CAKE:
1½ cups sugar
¾ cups all-purpose flour
6 tablespoons unsweetened cocoa powder
10 large egg whites

1½ teaspoons cream of tartar
¼ teaspoon fine sea salt or kosher salt
1½ teaspoons vanilla extract

FOR THE STRAWBERRIES:
3 pints fresh strawberries
6 tablespoons sugar
1½ tablespoons brandy

1. Preheat the oven to 350°F. To prepare the cake, sift ¾ cup sugar with the flour and cocoa and set aside.

2. In the bowl of a mixer fitted with the whisk attachment, beat the egg whites with the cream of tartar and salt until soft peaks form. Sprinkle the remaining sugar over the egg whites, 2 tablespoons at a time, beating after each addition. Beat until stiff peaks form. Fold in the vanilla extract. Gently but thoroughly fold in the sifted dry ingredients in three additions.

3. Pour the batter into an ungreased 10-inch angel food cake pan and bake until the cake is tall and lightly golden, and the top springs back when lightly touched, about 45 minutes. Cool the cake upside down by inverting the pan on a long neck bottle for 1½ hours. Slide a thin spatula around the sides and then the bottom of the cake to loosen it before turning it onto a plate. (The cake can be made two days ahead.)

4. Preheat the oven to 450°F.

5. In a bowl, combine the strawberries, sugar, and brandy. Spread the berries in a single layer on a rimmed baking sheet. Roast, tossing once, until the syrup is thick and bubbling, about 10 minutes. Let cool.

6. Preheat the broiler or use a toaster oven. Slice the cake gently with a serrated knife and toast or grill the slices on both sides.

7. Serve the cake with the strawberries, garnished with ice cream, sorbet, or crème fraîche.

☖MENU TWO (see page 84)

SEA SCALLOPS ON ROSEMARY SKEWERS WITH TOMATO-GINGER CHUTNEY

Roasted Asparagus with Scallions
Sea Scallops on Rosemary Skewers with Tomato-Ginger Chutney
Figs with Madeira and Orange Zest

ROASTED ASPARAGUS WITH SCALLIONS

Difficulty: Easy
Prep Time: 30 minutes
Cook Time: 15 minutes
Servings: 4

Waldy Says: Asparagus is just sexy to eat. Watching your partner eat each green stalk may also give you both some ideas. The vitamin K will stimulate your circulation. Light yet flavorful, the nuttiness of grilled asparagus is enhanced by the combination of soft melting cheese and crisp breadcrumbs. If you have some truffle oil in your pantry, use just a few drops to garnish.

1 bunch (about 1 pound) jumbo asparagus, bottoms trimmed, lower stalks peeled
2 tablespoons extra-virgin olive oil
½ teaspoon coarse sea salt or kosher salt, or more to taste
Freshly ground black pepper to taste
⅓ cup dried unseasoned breadcrumbs
2 scallions, minced
¼ cup grated Bel Paese or mild white cheddar cheese
Truffle oil, for garnish (optional)

1. Preheat the broiler. Toss the asparagus with the olive oil, salt, and pepper to taste.

2. Place the asparagus in the broiler, turning once, until they are browned and tender, about 10 to 12 minutes. Transfer the asparagus to an ovenproof gratin dish and set aside.

3. In a large frying pan over medium-high heat, toast the breadcrumbs until golden, stirring so they brown evenly, about 3 minutes. Put in a bowl and stir in the scallions and cheese.

4. Sprinkle the breadcrumb mixture over the asparagus and place the dish under the broiler until the topping is browned and crisp, about 1 minute. Divide the asparagus between four plates and garnish with a few drops of truffle oil if desired.

SEA SCALLOPS ON ROSEMARY SKEWERS WITH TOMATO-GINGER CHUTNEY

Difficulty: Medium
Prep Time: 30 minutes
Cook Time: 45 minutes
Servings: 4

Waldy Says: The scallops' caramelized flavor is offset by a bold chutney made spicy, with chili peppers, coriander, and cardamom, and a little sweet with candied ginger. The chutney can be prepared a few days in advance and kept in the refrigerator. The garlic and tomatoes are fabulous antioxidants.

FOR THE SEA SCALLOPS:

16 small branches rosemary
16 large sea scallops
4 tablespoons extra-virgin olive oil
Coarse sea salt or kosher salt to taste
Freshly ground black pepper to taste

FOR THE TOMATO-GINGER CHUTNEY:

½ cup finely chopped onion
2 garlic cloves, minced
2 jalapeno peppers, seeded and diced
2 teaspoons ground coriander
1 teaspoon mustard powder

½ teaspoon ground cardamom
½ cup dry white wine
5 large, ripe tomatoes, cored, seeded, and diced
1 cup finely chopped candied ginger
½ lemon, juiced

1. Strip enough leaves off each rosemary branch to make room for 1 scallop and coarsely chop the rosemary leaves. Thread the scallops horizontally onto the branches and lay them on a plate. Drizzle 2 tablespoons olive oil and the chopped rosemary leaves evenly over the scallops and season with salt and pepper. Turn gently to coat and let them sit at room temperature for 30 minutes.

2. Preheat the oven to 500°F or light the grill.

3. Meanwhile, prepare the tomato-ginger chutney. Warm 2 tablespoons of olive oil in a medium saucepan over medium heat. Add the onion and cook, stirring, until translucent, 3 to 4 minutes. Add the garlic, jalapeno, coriander, mustard powder, and cardamom, and cook for another minute. Add the wine and simmer for 2 minutes. Stir in the tomato and candied ginger and simmer until thick and jammy, about 20 to 30 minutes. Season with salt and pepper and cover to keep warm.

4. In the oven: Lay the scallop skewers on a rimmed baking sheet and roast until the scallops are opaque throughout, about 5 minutes. On the grill: Place the scallop skewers on the grill (or use a grilling basket), and cook, turning once, until the scallops are opaque throughout, about 5 minutes.

5. To serve, spread the tomato-ginger chutney on a serving dish. Arrange the scallops on top and sprinkle the lemon juice over all.

FIGS WITH MADEIRA AND ORANGE ZEST

Difficulty: Easy
Prep Time: 15 minutes
Cook Time: 20 minutes
Servings: 6

Waldy Says: If you have never had a grilled or roasted fig, I have a sexy surprise for you. Here I add Madeira, a fortified wine, and orange zest, which accents both the flavor of figs and the smoky flavors of roasting or grilling. The Madeira reduces into syrup that mixes with the red, portlike juices of the figs and fresh orange segments in this simple yet intense dessert.

2 oranges
1 cup sugar
½ cup Madeira
½ cup water
1 pint fresh figs
1 tablespoon extra-virgin olive oil,
    hazelnut oil, or walnut oil

1. Preheat the oven to 500°F. Using a vegetable peeler, remove the zest from half of one of the oranges.

2. In a small saucepan, combine the sugar, Madeira, orange zest, and water and bring to a boil, stirring occasionally. Simmer for 2 minutes, then turn off the heat and set aside.

3. Trim the stems from the figs and cut an X into their skins where the stems were. Place the figs in a dish or baking pan large enough to hold them snugly in one layer, and pour the syrup over them.

4. Place the baking pan with the figs in the oven and roast, basting occasionally, for 5 to 10 minutes. Turn the figs and roast until they are soft and the syrup has begun to thicken, another 3 to 5 minutes.

5. Cut the top and bottom off the oranges and stand them up on a cutting board on one of the flat sides. Using a small knife, cut away the peel and white pith, following the curve of the fruit, until the flesh is exposed. Cut the segments of fruit away from the membranes that connect them. Dice the segments, then place them in a bowl. Add the oil to the fruit and toss to combine.

6. To serve, spoon some of the oranges onto each dessert plate and arrange two or three figs beside them. Drizzle the oranges and figs with the Madeira syrup.

WEEK TWO

◖◖MENU ONE   (see page 117)

SUMMER VEGETABLE RISOTTO

Sweet Tomato and Mozzarella Salad
with Grilled Scallions
Summer Vegetable Risotto
Peaches with Balsamic Vinegar and Roquefort

SWEET TOMATO AND MOZZARELLA SALAD WITH GRILLED SCALLIONS

Difficulty: Easy
Prep Time: 30 minutes
Cook Time: 10 minutes
Servings: 4

Waldy Says: This is my robust revision of the popular Italian salad of sliced tomatoes, red onion, and mozzarella. This has green scallions and white cheese with a mix of red and yellow pear tomatoes. Combine for a great looking salad, and one full of foods to improve your circulation. Roasting the scallions softens them and brings out their sweetness.

2 bunches scallions, white and light green
    parts only (about 6 inches in length)
2½ tablespoons extra-virgin olive oil
Coarse sea salt or kosher salt to taste
Freshly ground black pepper to taste
1 pint pear, cherry, or grape tomatoes, halved
¾ pound fresh mozzarella, cut into
    diced-sized squares
¼ cup chopped fresh mint leaves

1. Light the broiler. Place the scallions in a large bowl and toss them with 1 tablespoon oil and season with salt and pepper.

2. Spread the scallions on a cookie sheet and cook, turning once, until they are charred yet still firm at their centers, about 6 minutes.

3. Let the scallions cool slightly, then slice them in half.

4. In a salad bowl, toss the scallions with the tomatoes, mozzarella, and mint. Drizzle with the remaining 1½ tablespoons of oil and season with salt and pepper.

⊚⁄ SUMMER VEGETABLE RISOTTO

Difficulty: Medium
Prep Time: 30 minutes
Cook Time: 15 minutes
Servings: 4

Waldy Says: Consider the recipe as just a guide—feel free to add other vegetables, like peppers or asparagus, or to use this as a formula for a single vegetable risotto using all zucchini, all eggplant, or whatever is most abundant.

2 small zucchini, sliced crosswise ¼-inch
    thick
2 small yellow squash, sliced crosswise
    ¼-inch thick
1 Japanese eggplant, sliced crosswise
    ¼-inch thick
3 tablespoons extra-virgin olive oil,
    plus more for brushing
Coarse sea salt or kosher salt to taste
Freshly ground black pepper to taste
1 large, ripe tomato, halved and seeded
1 tablespoon balsamic vinegar
5 to 6 cups vegetable or chicken broth
    (low-sodium if canned)
¼ cup minced shallots
1 large garlic clove, minced
2 cups Italian risotto rice, such as Arborio,
    Vialone, or Carnaroli
½ cup dry white wine

½ cup grated Parmesan cheese, plus additional
    for serving
¼ cup chopped fresh basil, plus sprigs for
    garnish

1. In a bowl, toss the zucchini, yellow squash, and eggplant slices with 2 tablespoons olive oil and a large pinch of salt and pepper. Brush the tomatoes all over with oil and season the cut sides with salt and pepper.

2. Lay the vegetables and tomatoes on the grill or a cookie sheet, placing the tomatoes skin side down. Grill or broil turning once, until charred and tender, about 10 to 15 minutes. Transfer the tomatoes to a cutting board. Transfer the other vegetables to a bowl and drizzle with half the balsamic vinegar.

3. When the tomatoes are cool enough to handle, remove the skins and dice them into ½-inch cubes. Drizzle with the remaining balsamic vinegar.

4. In a saucepan, bring the broth to a boil, and then reduce the heat to low and keep the broth just below a simmer.

5. In a large saucepan over medium heat, warm 1 tablespoon olive oil. Stir in the shallots and garlic and sauté until tender, about 3 minutes. Add the rice and cook, stirring, for 2 more minutes.

6. Pour the white wine into the pot and stir until it is absorbed. Add the broth, ½ cup at a time, stirring between each addition until the liquid is practically absorbed. After 20 minutes, taste a grain of rice. Continue to add broth and cook, if necessary, until the rice is tender and creamy, yet still slightly firm at the center. The total cooking time should be about 25 minutes. Stir in half the roasted vegetables, the cheese, and chopped basil, and season with salt and pepper. Remove from the heat.

7. Serve the risotto topped with the remaining vegetables and basil sprigs, and pass grated cheese alongside.

PEACHES WITH BALSAMIC VINEGAR AND ROQUEFORT

Difficulty: Medium
Prep Time: 30 minutes
Cook Time: 30 minutes
Servings: 4

Waldy Says: This sexy and bold-flavored dessert will lead to an evening of adventure after the flavors stimulate all of your senses. Roquefort cheese and vinegar may sound like odd ingredients for a dessert, but it's actually a winning combination when anchored by sweet, summer peaches. Cooking concentrates the peaches, and a little balsamic heightens their fruitiness, while the creaminess and bite of the cheese adds richness and takes this dessert off the beaten track. Serve this alone or with a crisp cookie—but not with ice cream—and it will surprise and delight.

1 cup sugar
⅔ cup water
½ vanilla bean, split
4 large ripe peaches, halved and pitted
⅓ cup balsamic vinegar
¾ cup sliced almonds
3 tablespoons Roquefort or other good
    quality blue cheese, crumbled

1. Preheat the oven to 500°F.

2. In a saucepan, combine the sugar, water, and the vanilla bean and bring to a boil, stirring occasionally until the sugar dissolves. Simmer for 2 minutes, then set aside.

3. Score the peach halves with an X mark on their skin sides. Put them in a large bowl and add the sugar syrup, vanilla bean, and balsamic vinegar. Toss to coat.

4. Arrange the peaches skin-side down in a single layer in a 9-by-13-inch roasting pan. Pour the balsamic syrup over the peaches and roast, basting once or twice, for 8 minutes. Turn the peaches over

and roast for another 5 to 10 minutes, until the peaches are soft and their skins look caramelized.

5. Place the almonds in a small pan with a heat-proof handle. Place the pan in the oven and toast the almonds, tossing them frequently, until they are golden and fragrant, about 3 to 5 minutes.

6. To serve, place two peaches, skin-side down, on each plate. Sprinkle with blue cheese, drizzle with more of the balsamic syrup, and garnish with the toasted almonds.

MENU TWO   (see page 117)

CHILI-RUBBED CHICKEN FINGERS WITH MOLASSES AND BRANDY SAUCE

Shrimp with Tomato Horseradish Salsa
Chili-Rubbed Chicken Fingers
with Molasses and Brandy Sauce
Caramelized Bananas with Blood Oranges,
Rum, and Spices

GRILLED SHRIMP WITH TOMATO HORSERADISH SALSA

Difficulty: Medium
Prep Time: 45 minutes
Cook Time: 10 minutes
Servings: 4

Waldy Says: This recipe has all the spicy, intense flavors of a cocktail sauce but without the sugary stickiness of ketchup. The bright salsa is filled with herbs, horseradish, citrus, and peppers, all designed to lighten your mood and increase your libido.

FOR THE SALSA:

2 large, ripe beefsteak tomatoes, cored and finely
    chopped
¼ cup minced red onion

3 scallions, white and light green parts only,
  thinly sliced

3 tablespoons prepared horseradish

2 tablespoons minced cilantro

1 teaspoon extra-virgin olive oil

½ jalapeno pepper, or more to taste,
  seeded and minced

Freshly squeezed lemon juice to taste

Dash of Tabasco sauce, or more to taste

Coarse sea salt or kosher salt to taste

Freshly ground black pepper to taste

FOR THE SHRIMP:

1 pound large shrimp (about 20), peeled
  and de-veined, tail-on

1 tablespoon prepared horseradish

1 teaspoon extra-virgin olive oil

Coarse sea salt or kosher salt to taste

Freshly ground black pepper to taste

Lemon wedges and lettuce leaves for serving

1. Light the grill or preheat the broiler.

2. Combine all the salsa ingredients in a bowl and set aside.

3. In a large bowl, toss the shrimp with the horseradish, olive oil, salt, and pepper.

4. Place the shrimp in a grilling basket or on soaked skewers and grill, turning once, until they are opaque and browned on the edges, about 3 to 5 minutes.

5. To serve, spoon some salsa in a mound in the center of each plate and top with shrimp. Arrange lemon wedges around the shrimp or use the salsa as a dip. Make a bed of lettuce leaves on a platter and place the shrimp on the lettuce. Serve the salsa alongside in a bowl, garnished with lemon wedges. Serve hot or at room temperature.

CHILI-RUBBED CHICKEN FINGERS WITH MOLASSES AND BRANDY SAUCE

Difficulty: Easy
Prep Time: 30 minutes
Cook Time: 15 minutes
Servings: 4 to 6 as a main course
             (about 30 skewers)

Waldy Says: Sweet and a little spicy, these satay-like skewers are a fun main course, or the perfect party hors d'oeuvres that your lover will love. Make sure to use fresh chili powder so they have some oomph. You will also get a little kick from the vitamin K in the molasses. If you plan to use wooden skewers, don't forget to soak them for at least an hour before cooking.

3½ pounds boneless, skinless chicken breasts

1 tablespoon ground cumin

1 tablespoon chili powder

½ teaspoon coarse sea salt or kosher salt,
  plus additional to taste

Freshly ground black pepper to taste

½ cup light molasses

3 tablespoons brandy

2 bunches scallions, trimmed and sliced
  into 6-inch lengths

1 tablespoon extra-virgin olive oil

1. Rinse the chicken and pat dry with paper towels. Cut the chicken breasts lengthwise into ½-inch thick strips.

2. In a medium bowl, combine the cumin, chili powder, salt, and a good amount of pepper. Add the chicken breast strips and toss until thoroughly coated. Cover the bowl with plastic wrap and refrigerate for at least 1 hour, and preferably 4 hours or overnight.

3. Preheat the broiler. Thread the chicken strips onto skewers using one skewer per strip. In a small saucepan, bring the molasses and brandy to a boil, stirring. Brush the chicken all over with the molasses-brandy glaze.

4. Put the scallions in a bowl and toss them with the olive oil and a pinch of salt and pepper.

5. Spread the scallions on a pan and place it four inches away from the heat source. Broil until browned and tender, about 2½ minutes. Remove from the oven and tent with foil to keep warm. Put the skewered chicken in a pan and broil, turning once, until it is cooked through and browned around the edges, about 3 minutes.

6. Serve the chicken with the scallions, drizzling additional molasses-brandy glaze over all.

CARAMELIZED BANANAS WITH BLOOD ORANGES, RUM, AND SPICES

Difficulty: Medium
Prep Time: 30 minutes
Cook Time: 15 minutes
Servings: 6

Waldy Says: In this luscious dessert, roasted bananas are caramelized with brown sugar, and spices and blood oranges add another dimension to what can otherwise be an overly round, sweet flavor. Serve this as is with a little sour cream. Magnesium and potassium in the bananas combine with the vitamin C in the blood oranges to provide a hidden bonus of increased blood flow.

3 small blood oranges
¼ cup dark rum
1 teaspoon whole allspice
2 whole cloves
¼ cup dark brown sugar, packed
1 tablespoon unsalted butter
1 tablespoon freshly squeezed lemon juice
¼ teaspoon freshly ground black pepper
4 ripe bananas, peeled, halved lengthwise
    then crosswise into quarters
¼ teaspoon ground cinnamon

⅛ teaspoon freshly grated nutmeg
Sour cream, for serving

1. Preheat the broiler and position a rack 6 inches from the heat source. Squeeze two of the blood oranges and strain the juice (you should have ¼ cup of juice).

2. In a saucepan over medium heat, combine the orange juice, rum, allspice, and cloves and bring to a boil. Simmer for 5 minutes, then add the sugar and continue to simmer, stirring until the sugar dissolves and the mixture is syrupy, about 5 minutes. Stir in the butter, lemon juice, black pepper, cinnamon, and nutmeg.

3. Cut the top and bottom off the third orange and stand it up on a cutting board on one of its flat sides. Using a small knife, cut away the peel and white pith, following the curve of the fruit, until the flesh is exposed. Working over a bowl, cut the segments of fruit away from the membranes, letting the fruit and juices fall into the bowl.

4. Lay the bananas in a pan just large enough to accommodate them in a single layer. Strain the rum sauce over them and then scatter the orange segments and juice over all. Broil, basting frequently with the pan juices, until the bananas are soft and the juices are thick and browned, about 5 to 7 minutes. Serve with dollops of sour cream.

WEEK THREE

MENU ONE   (see page 133)

TURKEY PAILLARDS WITH BLACK PEPPER, SAGE, AND GARLIC

Spicy Potato Salad with Sweet and Hot Peppers
Turkey Paillards with Black Pepper,
Sage, and Garlic
Grilled Pineapple with Gin, Juniper, and Lime

SPICY POTATO SALAD WITH SWEET AND HOT PEPPERS

Difficulty:　Medium
Prep Time:　45 minutes
Cook Time:　30 minutes
Servings:　4

Waldy Says: Mayo-free, this dish could not be further from your mom's potato salad. The grilled potatoes are smoky and assertive enough to match the intensity of the grilled chilies and sweet bell peppers they're tossed with, not to mention the addition of capers and anchovies. All the flavors pack a spicy Mediterranean punch making these potatoes very sexy and bold. If you don't like anchovies, just leave them out.

1¾ pounds small red potatoes, scrubbed and quartered
4 tablespoons extra-virgin olive oil, plus additional to brush the peppers
Coarse sea salt or kosher salt to taste
Freshly ground black pepper to taste
1 red bell pepper
1 green bell pepper
1 hot chili pepper such as Serrano, Thai Chile, or Scotch Bonnet
1½ tablespoons red wine vinegar
2 scallions, finely chopped
¼ cup chopped black Moroccan oil-cured pitted olives
2 anchovies, chopped (optional)
2 tablespoons flat leaf parsley, chopped, for garnish
Lettuce leaves, for serving

1. Preheat the broiler. In a large bowl, toss the potatoes with 2 tablespoons of the olive oil and season generously with salt and pepper.
2. Halve the bell peppers and hot pepper lengthwise. Seed and stem them, then spread, skin side up, on a baking sheet. Lightly brush the pepper skins with olive oil. Broil the peppers as close to the heat source as possible, until well charred, about 5 minutes. Immediately transfer the peppers to a large bowl and cover with a plate. Let steam for 5 minutes. Turn the broiler off and preheat the oven to 500°F.
3. Spread the potatoes in a single layer on a rimmed baking sheet and roast, turning every 5 minutes, until crisp on the outside and cooked through, about 20 minutes.
4. Remove the peel from the peppers using a spoon or your fingers. (Make sure to wear gloves while working with the chili pepper.) Chop the peppers into ½-inch pieces.
5. In a small bowl, whisk together vinegar, scallions, and salt and pepper to taste. Whisking constantly, drizzle in the remaining 2 tablespoons olive oil. In a large bowl, toss the warm potatoes with the peppers and enough of the dressing to coat the vegetables. Gently mix in the olives and anchovies. Taste and add more dressing and/or salt and pepper if desired. Garnish with parsley and serve warm or at room temperature on lettuce leaves.

TURKEY PAILLARDS WITH BLACK PEPPER, SAGE, AND GARLIC

Difficulty:　Easy
Prep Time:　30 minutes
Cook Time:　10 minutes
Servings:　4

Waldy Says: The garlic, capers, sage, and lemon should stimulate more than just your taste buds. These turkey breasts are so thin that they cook in a flash. You can buy thin turkey cutlets precut, or simply slice turkey breasts into cutlets, pounding them to an even thickness if you like. The marinade of garlic, pepper, and sage makes them particularly savory, reminiscent of deconstructed turkey with sage stuffing. Get the rest of the meal ready to go before you grill or broil these, since overcooking will rob them of their succulence.

8 boneless, skinless turkey breasts,
    sliced ½-inch thick, 4 ounces each
½ cup extra-virgin olive oil
4 garlic cloves, thinly sliced
3 tablespoons chopped, fresh sage
Coarse sea salt or kosher salt to taste
Freshly ground black pepper to taste
2 tablespoons capers, drained, for garnish
8 lemon wedges, for garnish

1. Rinse the turkey and pat dry with paper towels. Combine the olive oil, garlic, sage, and a pinch of salt and pepper in a wide, shallow bowl. Mix together using the back of a fork to crush the garlic a bit and blend the flavors. Add the turkey breasts to the marinade and turn to coat. Cover the bowl and let sit at room temperature for 30 minutes, or refrigerate for 2 hours or overnight.

2. Preheat the broiler.

3. Lay the turkey under the broiler and cook, turning once, until well seared and done in the center, about 5 to 6 minutes.

4. Serve sprinkled with capers and garnished with lemon wedges.

GRILLED PINEAPPLE WITH GIN, JUNIPER, AND LIME

Difficulty: Easy
Prep Time: 15 minutes
Cook Time: 15 minutes
Servings: 4 to 6

Waldy Says: I was probably served a Hawaiian version of a gin and tonic garnished with pineapple at some point in my life, or else I just made up this gin-flavored dessert. The piney, earthy flavor of juniper is a nice foil to the bright acidity of the pineapple and lime, and the effect is refreshing and simple, yet very flavorful, and it should get your juices flowing.

Juniper berries are not hard to find (see below), but the dish is worth making even if you don't have them.

1 lime
½ cup, plus 2 tablespoons sugar
2 tablespoons water
¼ cup gin
5 juniper berries, lightly crushed (see note)
1 vanilla bean, split lengthwise, pulp scraped
1 ripe pineapple, peeled and trimmed
Vanilla ice cream and/or berry or tropical
    fruit sorbet, for serving

1. Light the grill. Grate the zest from the lime and then juice it.

2. In a saucepan over medium heat, combine ½ cup sugar, water, the lime zest and juice, gin, juniper berries, and vanilla bean. Bring to a simmer, stirring until the sugar dissolves. Simmer until thickened, about 5 minutes.

3. Core the pineapple if desired and cut it crosswise into ½-inch rounds. Sprinkle the pineapple slices with the remaining 2 tablespoons of sugar on both sides, then use tongs to carefully lay them on the grill. Cook, turning once, until caramelized, about 5 to 8 minutes per side.

4. Transfer the pineapple slices to a platter and pour the lime syrup over them. Serve with ice cream and/or sorbet.

NOTE: Juniper berries are available in many supermarkets, or you can mail order them from Penzeys Spices, 1-800-741-7787.

◖◗MENU TWO   (see page 133)

HALIBUT WITH LEMON CONFIT AND WHITE WINE

Seared Filet Mignon Tartare
Halibut with Lemon Confit and White Wine
Individual Warm Chocolate Cake with
Roasted Apricots

◉ SEARED FILET MIGNON TARTARE

Difficulty: Easy-Medium
Prep Time: 45 minutes
Cook Time: 10 minutes
Servings: 4

Waldy Says: The flavors, pungency, and texture of this dish will give you an energy and mood boost. This is a twist on the classic tartare of chopped raw beef. Here I add another level of flavor by searing the outside of the steak to create a great smokiness, while the inside remains raw. It's worth the time to chop the steak by hand with a really sharp knife or in a meat grinder (either the old fashioned kind or with a meat grinding attachment on a mixer) to give it a nice texture—a food processor will make it pasty. The meat is seasoned with the intense flavors of red onion, mustard, and capers, and you can serve more of these ingredients on the side as garnishes.

2 8-ounce filet mignons, trimmed
Coarse sea salt or kosher salt to taste
Freshly ground black pepper to taste
1 tablespoon extra-virgin olive oil
2 tablespoons Dijon-style mustard
1 tablespoon chopped capers, plus
    additional whole capers for garnish
2 anchovy fillets, minced
1 tablespoon minced red onion, plus
    additional chopped red onion for garnish

2 teaspoons Worcestershire sauce
½ teaspoon freshly squeezed lemon juice
6 dashes Tabasco, or to taste
2 cups baby salad greens, washed and spun dry
Cracked fresh black peppercorns, for garnish

1. Preheat the broiler. Generously season the filet mignons with salt and pepper and drizzle them with olive oil.

2. Place the filets on a baking sheet and position it directly under the heat source. Broil the meat until it is charred on all sides, about 2 minutes for the top and bottom plus another minute or two for the sides.

3. Let the filets cool thoroughly. Wrap them in plastic and refrigerate until cold, at least 2 hours.

4. Chop the meat finely or grind in a meat grinder and place in a large bowl. Season the meat with generous grindings of black pepper. Add the mustard, capers, anchovy, red onion, Worcestershire sauce, lemon juice, and Tabasco. Taste and add additional salt if desired.

5. Place the baby greens on a platter and mound the tartare over the greens. Garnish with the capers, red onion, and cracked peppercorns.

◉ HALIBUT WITH LEMON CONFIT AND WHITE WINE

Difficulty: Medium
Prep Time: 30 minutes
Cook Time: 1 hour
Servings: 4

Waldy Says: This dish will provide you with energy for endurance and agility. The lightness of the fish and lemon will leave you satisfied but not bloated. This simple dish gets its bright flavor from a simmered, jammy lemon confit that is both tart and slightly sweet. Leftover lemon confit can be used in myriad ways—try it on broiled scallops, or use it as a marinade for grilled shrimp.

3 lemons
1 cup dry white wine
3 tablespoons sugar
1 teaspoon fresh thyme leaves, plus additional sprigs
1 teaspoon freshly ground black pepper, plus additional to taste
¼ teaspoon coarse sea salt or kosher salt, plus additional to taste
4 halibut fillets, skin on (1-inch thick)
Extra-virgin olive oil
Watercress sprigs, for garnish

1. Slice two of the lemons in half lengthwise, then thinly slice into half-moons. Slice the remaining lemon into thin rounds. Reserve the rounds.

2. Place the half-moons of lemons, wine, sugar, thyme leaves, pepper, and salt in a saucepan and bring to a boil over medium heat. Cover and simmer until the lemons are soft, about 10 minutes. Uncover and cook slowly until the liquid has a syrupy consistency, about 25 to 30 minutes more. Let cool.

3. Preheat the oven to 450°F. Transfer the lemons and their liquid to the bowl of a food processor and pulse until finely chopped (do not let them become a purée). You can also finely chop the lemons by hand.

4. Brush the skin sides of the halibut fillets with olive oil and place, skin side down, on a rimmed baking sheet. Season the fillets with salt and pepper, then spread the tops and sides of each fillet with the lemon confit. Scatter the thyme sprigs over the fillets and top with the reserved lemon rounds.

5. Place the pan in the oven and roast until the fish is opaque throughout, about 10 minutes.

6. Serve the fillets with the watercress sprigs.

INDIVIDUAL WARM CHOCOLATE CAKES WITH ROASTED APRICOTS

Difficulty: Medium
Prep Time: 30 minutes
Cook Time: 15 minutes
Servings: 2 individual cakes

Waldy Says: Warm and fluffy outside, warm and gooey inside, like a fallen soufflé, this dessert will elicit more sensory exploration.

2 ounces butter, plus a little more for buttering the molds
2 ounces bittersweet chocolate, preferably Valhrona
1 egg
1 egg yolk
2 tablespoons sugar
1 teaspoon cake or all-purpose flour, plus a little more for dusting.

1. Preheat oven to 450°F. Using a double boiler, heat the butter and chocolate together until the chocolate is almost melted. While that is heating, beat the egg, yolk, and sugar together with a whisk or electric beater until light and thick. The melted chocolate and butter should be quite warm; beat together. Pour in the egg mixture, then quickly beat in the flour, just until combined.

2. Butter and lightly flour two 4-ounce molds, custard cups or ramekins. Tap out excess flour. Divide the batter among the molds. At this point you can refrigerate the desserts until you are ready to eat. Bring them back to room temperature before cooking.

3. Place the molds on a tray and bake for 6 to 7 minutes; the center will be quite soft, but the sides will be set. Invert each mold onto a plate and let sit for about 10 seconds. Unmold by lifting up one corner of the mold; the cakes will fall out onto the plate. Serve immediately.

> ## THE HARDNESS FACTOR
> ### HALFWAY MILESTONE DINNER
> (see page 134)
>
> ### PEPPERED TUNA WITH RED WINE AND SHALLOTS
>
> Chilled Yellow Tomato Soup
> Peppered Tuna with Red Wine and Shallots
> Peaches with Balsamic Vinegar and Roquefort

CHILLED YELLOW TOMATO SOUP

Difficulty: Medium
Prep Time: 45 minutes
Cook Time: 45 minutes
Servings: 6

Waldy Says: The tomatoes, peppers, herbs, and spices will excite all your senses. Make this soup a day ahead.

FOR THE SOUP:

6 large yellow tomatoes
2½ tablespoons extra-virgin olive oil
1 teaspoon coarse sea salt or kosher salt,
    plus additional to taste
1 cup chopped onion
2 garlic cloves, minced
1 teaspoon whole coriander seed
½ teaspoon whole cumin seed
1½ cups water
1 tablespoon fresh lemon juice
½ teaspoon freshly ground black pepper

FOR THE CILANTRO-ONION RELISH:

1 medium red tomato, seeded and diced
½ cup finely chopped red onion
¼ cup chopped cilantro
1 tablespoon fresh lime juice
1 tablespoon extra-virgin olive oil
1 teaspoon minced jalapeno
Coarse sea salt or kosher salt to taste
Freshly ground black pepper to taste

1. Light the grill or preheat the oven to 500°F. Place the tomatoes in a bowl and toss them with 1½ tablespoons olive oil and salt to taste.

2. On the grill: Place the whole tomatoes on the grill for 10 to 15 minutes, turning until the tomatoes are charred. In the oven: Place the whole tomatoes in a roasting pan and roast for 10 minutes. Turn the tomatoes over and roast for another 5 minutes.

3. Transfer the tomatoes to a bowl and let cool slightly. Core and roughly chop them, reserving their juices. Heat the remaining tablespoon of oil in a large pot over medium heat. Add the onions and garlic and cook, stirring, until they are translucent, about 5 minutes. Do not let them brown (if they start to color, add a tablespoon of water).

4. Meanwhile, in a small skillet, toast the coriander and cumin over medium-high heat until they are fragrant and lightly browned, shaking the pan so the spices don't burn, about 2 minutes. Add them to the pot, along with the tomatoes and their liquid, and water. Stir in 1 teaspoon salt.

5. Bring the tomato mixture to a boil over high heat, then reduce the heat and simmer for about 15 minutes.

6. Turn off the heat and let the soup cool slightly. Purée the soup either with an immersion blender, or in batches in a blender or food processor. Strain through a coarse sieve and discard the solids. Chill the soup until cold, at least 4 hours.

7. Season soup with lemon juice, salt to taste, and pepper.

8. Meanwhile, in a bowl, stir together all the ingredients for the cilantro-onion relish.

9. Serve soup garnished with a spoonful of the cilantro-onion relish.

℗ PEPPERED TUNA WITH RED WINE AND SHALLOTS

Difficulty:	Medium-Difficult
Prep Time:	45 minutes
Cook Time:	30 minutes
Servings:	4

Waldy Says: This sexy fish dish provides you with all of the energy required for optimum performance. Serve it with watercress salad and potatoes.

4 tuna steaks (1¼ inches thick)
Coarse sea salt or kosher salt to taste
2 teaspoons very coarsely ground black pepper
1 cup dry red wine
½ cup port
3 shallots, diced (about ¾ cup)
1 cup cherry tomatoes, halved
2 teaspoons extra-virgin olive oil
Basil sprigs, for garnish (optional)

1. Season the tuna steaks with salt on both sides, then pat the pepper all over them. Wrap in plastic and refrigerate for 1 hour.

2. In a saucepan over medium heat, combine the wine, port, and shallots and bring to a boil. Simmer until syruplike and reduced, about 20 minutes. Keep warm.

3. Position a well-seasoned or lightly oiled cast-iron skillet 6 inches from the heat source and preheat the broiler for 10 minutes. You can also use an oiled, heavy-duty baking pan. Or, light the grill.

4. In the oven: Carefully lay the tuna steaks in the preheated pan and broil until charred around the edges, about 2 minutes. Turn and cook for 2 minutes more for rare, or until done to taste. On the grill: Lightly oil the grill or a grilling basket. Place the tuna on the grill (or use the basket) and cook for 2 to 3 minutes per side for rare, or until done to taste.

5. In a bowl, toss the cherry tomatoes with the olive oil and season with salt and pepper. Use a slotted spoon to mound the shallots on a platter, top with the tuna, and surround with the tomatoes. Drizzle with the red wine–port syrup and garnish with basil sprigs if desired.

℗ PEACHES WITH BALSAMIC VINEGAR AND ROQUEFORT

Difficulty:	Medium
Prep Time:	30 minutes
Cook Time:	30 minutes
Servings:	4

Waldy Says: Get ready for an evening of adventure after these flavors excite all of your senses. Serve as is or with a crisp cookie for a delightful taste surprise.

4 large ripe peaches, halved and pitted
1 cup sugar
⅔ cup water
½ vanilla bean, split
⅓ cup balsamic vinegar
¾ cup sliced almonds
3 tablespoons Roquefort or other
    good quality blue cheese, crumbled

1. Preheat the oven to 500°F.

2. In a saucepan, combine the sugar, water, and the vanilla bean and bring to a boil, stirring occasionally until the sugar dissolves. Simmer for 2 minutes, then set aside.

3. Score the peach halves with an X mark on their skin sides. Put them in a large bowl and add the sugar syrup, vanilla bean, and balsamic vinegar. Toss to coat.

4. Arrange the peaches skin-side down in a single layer in a 9-by-13-inch roasting pan. Pour the balsamic syrup over the peaches and roast, basting once or twice, for 8 minutes. Turn the peaches over and roast for another 5 to 10 minutes, until the peaches are soft and their skins look caramelized.

5. Place the almonds in a small pan with a heat-proof handle. Place the pan in the oven and toast the almonds, tossing them frequently, until they are golden and fragrant, about 3 to 5 minutes.

6. To serve, place two peaches, skin-side down, on each plate. Sprinkle with blue cheese, drizzle with more of the balsamic syrup, and garnish with the toasted almonds.

WEEK FOUR

┌─────────────────────────────────────┐

⟨☾MENU ONE   (see page 167)

ROASTED SHELLFISH STEW WITH TOMATOES AND GARLIC

Mediterranean Stuffed Zucchini with
Cilantro-Yogurt Sauce
Roasted Shellfish Stew with Tomatoes
and Garlic
Almond Ricotta Cake with Moscato
Roasted Apricots

└─────────────────────────────────────┘

⟨☾ MEDITERRANEAN STUFFED ZUCCHINI WITH CILANTRO-YOGURT SAUCE

Difficulty: Medium-Difficult
Prep Time: 1 hour
Cook Time: 30 minutes
Servings: 6

Waldy Says: This is a great side dish, appetizer, or vegetarian main course. The spices, herbs, and even the shape will inspire great success at the dinner table and in bed.

3 garlic cloves
3 medium zucchini, trimmed
3 tablespoons extra-virgin olive oil
1 small onion, chopped
2 tablespoons chopped fresh cilantro

2 tablespoons chopped fresh mint
1/8 teaspoon ground cumin
1 teaspoon coarse sea salt or kosher salt,
    plus additional to taste
1 teaspoon freshly ground black pepper,
    plus additional to taste
3 tablespoons plain dried breadcrumbs
1 cup plain yogurt
2 tablespoons milk or cream
Lemon wedges, for serving

1. Preheat the oven to 500°F.

2. Finely chop two of the garlic cloves. Cut off one quarter of each zucchini at the stem end, chop this finely, and set aside. Halve the remaining part of the zucchinis lengthwise, and scoop out the seeded flesh to form zucchini boats with 1/4-inch thick walls. Chop the scooped out zucchini and add it to the reserved chopped zucchini.

3. In a pan, warm 1 tablespoon oil over medium heat. Add the onion and the chopped garlic and cook, stirring, until the onion is translucent, about 10 minutes. Add the chopped zucchini, 1 tablespoon each of the cilantro and mint, and the cumin. Season with 3/4 teaspoon salt and the pepper, and cook, stirring for another 3 minutes. Transfer to a bowl and let cool slightly. Stuff the zucchini boats with this mixture.

4. Place the stuffed zucchini in a baking dish just large enough to hold them. Sprinkle the breadcrumbs over them, drizzle with 2 tablespoons oil, and season with salt and pepper. Roast until the breadcrumb topping is browned, about 12 minutes.

5. Meanwhile, place the yogurt in a bowl and stir it with a whisk to loosen it. Whisk in the cream or milk. Add the remaining tablespoon each of cilantro and mint. Using the side of a chef's knife, or a mortar and pestle, mash the remaining garlic clove with 1/4 teaspoon salt to form a paste. Whisk the garlic purée into the yogurt. Serve the zucchini hot, drizzled with the sauce and a squeeze of lemon if desired.

ROASTED SHELLFISH STEW WITH TOMATOES AND GARLIC

Difficulty: Medium-Difficult
Prep Time: 45 minutes
Cook Time: 30 minutes
Servings: 4

Waldy Says: This exuberant seafood stew has the same spectacular impact as its Mediterranean relatives bouillabaisse and paella, but it's also much easier to prepare since everything goes in the pot at once. Thinly sliced Idaho potatoes cook in the soup and their starch thickens the broth, while linguica sausage adds spice and richness. I like to use shell-on shrimp since it's meant to be a rustic, roll-up-your-sleeves kind of dish. Feed each other, eat with your hands, and make a mess. Who knows where you will end up?

16 cherrystone or topneck clams
32 mussels, debearded
1 tablespoon extra-virgin olive oil
16 jumbo shrimp, de-veined, shells on
½ Spanish onion, chopped (about 1 cup)
3 garlic cloves, chopped
6 small red bliss or fingerling potatoes, scrubbed, halved, and thinly sliced
2 large, ripe tomatoes, cored and diced
½ teaspoon crushed red pepper flakes
½ cup dry white wine
2 cups chicken or vegetable broth (low-sodium if canned)
3 tablespoons chopped fresh flat-leaf parsley, for garnish

1. Preheat the oven to 500°F. Wash the clams and mussels in a bowl of cold water, changing the water several times. Discard any open shellfish that don't close when tapped.
2. In a flameproof, ovenproof casserole or very large skillet over high heat, warm the olive oil. Add the shrimp and cook, stirring, until the shells are slightly browned, about 2 minutes. Transfer shrimp to a plate and set aside.
3. Add the onion to olive oil and sauté until translucent, about 3 minutes. Add the garlic and continue to cook for 1 minute longer. Stir in the potatoes, tomatoes, and red pepper flakes. Pour in the wine and bring to a simmer. Let cook for 30 seconds. Add the broth and stir in the shrimp, clams, and mussels.
4. Place the casserole in the oven and roast until the clams and mussels have opened, about 15 to 20 minutes. Serve garnished with the parsley.

ALMOND RICOTTA CAKE WITH MOSCATO ROASTED APRICOTS

Difficulty: Medium
Prep Time: 45 minutes
Cook Time: 1 hour 15 minutes
Servings: 12

Waldy Says: Almond flavors always work well with stone fruits, in this case apricots. This country-style almond cake has a light, delicate texture and a moist creaminess that comes from the addition of ricotta cheese. Moscato, a perfumed sweet wine, reduces and combines with the juice of roasted apricots, giving the dessert an intense fragrance and elegance. Leftover apricots are also excellent served over ice cream or yogurt.

FOR THE CAKE:
¾ cup (1½ sticks) unsalted butter, melted and cooled, plus more for cake pan
Flour (all-purpose) for cake pan
1 cup sugar
1 teaspoon almond extract
Pinch of fine sea salt or kosher salt
4 large eggs
½ cup almond flour (see note)
1 teaspoon baking powder
Whipped cream or ice cream for serving

FOR THE APRICOTS:

1⅔ cups Moscato or other white dessert wine
  (1 375-milliliter bottle)
½ cup, plus 2 tablespoons sugar
1 teaspoon freshly squeezed lemon juice
1 pound ripe apricots (about 6 to 8), quartered
  and pitted
2 tablespoons unsalted butter,
  cut into pieces

1. Preheat oven to 350°F.

2. To prepare the cake, butter and flour a 10-inch cake pan and line it with parchment or wax paper. In the bowl of an electric mixer fitted with the whisk attachment, combine the butter, sugar, ricotta cheese, almond extract, and salt.

3. Beat at medium speed for 5 minutes. Add the eggs, one at a time, beating after each addition until fully incorporated. In a small bowl, whisk together the flour and baking powder, then fold into batter.

4. Scrape the batter into the prepared cake pan and bake for 30 to 35 minutes, until a tester inserted into the center of the cake comes out clean. Let cool thoroughly before removing from the pan.

5. To prepare the apricots, in a saucepan over medium heat, combine the Moscato, ½ cup sugar, and lemon juice, and bring to a simmer, stirring until the sugar is dissolved. Simmer until the liquid is reduced and syrupy, about 12 to 15 minutes.

6. Meanwhile, to roast the apricots, preheat the oven to 500°F. Spread the apricot halves in a single layer on a rimmed baking sheet, dot them with butter, and sprinkle with the remaining 2 tablespoons sugar. Roast until they begin to brown, about 8 to 10 minutes. Pour the Moscato syrup over the apricots and return to the oven for 10 minutes, until they are tender.

7. To serve, cut wedges of the cake and garnish with apricots, a drizzle of Moscato syrup, and whipped cream or ice cream.

NOTE: You can order almond flour from the King Arthur Flour Baker's Catalogue, 1-800-827-6836. Alternatively, to make your own almond flour, place ½ cup plus 1 tablespoon blanched sliced almonds in the bowl of a food processor with 3 tablespoons of flour from the recipe and process until the almonds are the same consistency of coarse meal. Stir well, being sure to get into the corners, and continue to process until finely ground (do not overprocess or the mixture will become pasty and unusable).

MENU TWO   (see page 167)

CRISP PENNE WITH RICOTTA, TOMATOES, AND HERBS

Roasted Clams with Garlic, Lemon,
and Red Pepper
Crisp Penne with Ricotta, Tomatoes, and Herbs
Lemon Pudding Cakes with Persimmon

ROASTED CLAMS WITH GARLIC, LEMON, AND RED PEPPER

Difficulty: Medium
Prep Time: 45 minutes
Cook Time: 15 minutes
Servings: 4 as a main course

Waldy Says: Simple Clams Casino to slurp, done with your hands. I have added ingredients that will stimulate your heart, taste buds, and libido.

1½ cups fresh breadcrumbs
¾ cup thinly sliced red bell pepper
  (about ½ a large pepper)
6 garlic cloves, thinly sliced
1 teaspoon freshly ground black pepper
Coarse sea salt or kosher salt to taste
1 lemon, halved lengthwise, thinly sliced
  (discard ends)

¼ cup extra-virgin olive oil
24 live topneck clams, scrubbed well in
    cold water
3 tablespoons chopped fresh mint,
    for garnish

1. Preheat the oven to 500°F.

2. In a large bowl, toss together the bread-crumbs, red peppers, garlic, black pepper, and salt. Gently squeeze the lemon slices over the bowl, then add them and toss well. Drizzle the olive oil over all and toss to combine.

3. Lay the clams on a baking pan in a single layer, with their lips facing up. Sprinkle the breadcrumb mixture over and around them. Roast until the clams open, about 10 to 12 minutes. Serve garnished with mint.

ᦡ CRISP PENNE WITH RICOTTA, TOMATOES, AND HERBS

Difficulty: Easy
Prep Time: 10 minutes
Cook Time: 30 minutes
Servings: 4

Waldy Says: This easy pasta dish can be prepared ahead of time so that you can focus on your date and task. Light yet satisfying enough to hold you through an entire evening.

Coarse sea salt or kosher salt to taste
1 pound penne pasta
2 pounds plum tomatoes (about 10 to 12),
    halved lengthwise
2 tablespoons extra-virgin olive oil
Freshly ground black pepper to taste
1¼ cups fresh ricotta cheese
¼ cup plus 1 tablespoon lowfat sour cream
¼ cup, plus 2 tablespoons grated Bel Paese
    cheese

¼ cup, plus 2 tablespoons grated Asiago cheese
1 tablespoon chopped fresh flat leaf parsley
2 tablespoons chopped fresh oregano or
    marjoram or a combination

1. Preheat the oven to 500°F. Bring a large pot of salted water to boil. Cook the penne in the boiling water until it is just barely al dente.

2. Lay the tomatoes cut side down on a rimmed baking sheet, drizzle them with the olive oil, and season them with salt and pepper. Place the baking sheet in the oven and roast until the tomatoes are soft and their skins are browned and peeling, about 10 minutes.

3. Lower temperature to 400°F. When the tomatoes are cool enough to handle, remove their skins and chop them. In a bowl, whisk together the ricotta and all the sour cream. In a large bowl, toss the drained penne with the ricotta mixture, then stir in ¼ cup each of the Bel Paese and Asiago cheeses. Mix in the herbs and season with salt and pepper.

4. Add half the tomatoes to the pasta and toss. Spread the pasta mixture in a 9-by-13-inch baking dish or large gratin dish and top with the remaining tomatoes. Sprinkle with the remaining 2 tablespoons each of Bel Paese and Asiago and additional black pepper to taste. Bake until the top is crisped, about 15 minutes. Serve immediately, while hot.

ᦡ LEMON PUDDING CAKES WITH PERSIMMON

Difficulty: Medium
Prep Time: 30 minutes
Cook Time: 45 minutes
Servings: 8

Waldy Says: Simultaneously tart and sweet, with great mouth "feel"—perhaps just like your lover.

¼ cup unsalted butter
1 cup plus 2 tablespoons sugar

Pinch of salt

3 tablespoons lemon zest

6 egg yolks

6 tablespoons flour

½ cup freshly squeezed lemon juice

2 cups milk

8 egg whites

3 ripe persimmons, peeled

3 tablespoons sugar

1. Preheat oven to 325°F.

2. To make the pudding cakes: Cream the butter, sugar, salt, and lemon zest. Add the egg yolks one at a time, mixing well after each addition. Add the flour and mix well. Add ¼ cup of the lemon juice and milk and mix until combined.

3. Beat the egg whites until they are stiff peaks and fold into the batter.

4. Immediately pour the batter into a plastic wrap–lined 9-by-13-inch pan and bake in a water bath at 325°F for 35 to 45 minutes, or until golden brown and firm. Refrigerate to chill for 2 hours or overnight. Invert onto a sheet pan. Cut out eight 3-inch squares just prior to serving.

5. Prepare the persimmons: Slice two of the persimmons into ⅛-inch wedges and set aside.

6. Prepare the persimmon sauce: Purée the remaining persimmon with the remaining ¼ cup lemon juice and the sugar for 2 minutes or until smooth. Strain through a fine mesh sieve and thin with a little water, if necessary.

7. Place a circle of cake in the center of each plate and arrange the persimmon slices on top in a pinwheel. Drizzle the persimmon sauce around the plates.

WEEK FIVE

MENU ONE   (see page 189)

PEPPERED TUNA WITH RED WINE AND SHALLOTS

Seared Polenta Squares with Spicy Broccoli Rabe
Peppered Tuna with Red Wine and Shallots
Raspberry Cake

SEARED POLENTA SQUARES WITH SPICY BROCCOLI RABE

Difficulty: Medium
Prep Time: 2 days
Cook Time
    Day 1:   10 minutes
    Day 2:   20 minutes
Servings: 6

Waldy Says: Squares of firm cornmeal polenta really benefit from a quick sear in the oven. The squares crisp and caramelize at the edges, while the centers remain soft and creamy. Here, I top them with a spicy, slightly bitter sauté of broccoli rabe and plenty of garlic, and a shower of grated mozzarella cheese. It's a terrific combination of flavors, and it makes a very substantial side dish. In fact, this recipe could also serve as the main attraction for any vegetarians at the table (just remember to cook the polenta in vegetable broth or water!).

4 cups chicken or vegetable broth
    (low-sodium if canned), or water

1 cup instant polenta (see note, below)

1½ cups grated Parmesan cheese

½ teaspoon coarse sea salt or kosher salt,
    plus additional to taste

¼ teaspoon freshly ground black pepper,
    plus additional to taste

1½ pounds broccoli rabe, trimmed
3 tablespoons extra-virgin olive oil
3 garlic cloves, thinly sliced
1½ teaspoons red pepper flakes,
  or to taste
½ cup water
1 cup grated fresh mozzarella cheese
  (about 4 ounces)

1. Bring the broth to a boil in a medium saucepan. Turn the heat down to medium and add the polenta in a thin stream, stirring constantly with a whisk. Continue cooking, whisking all the while, until the polenta is quite thick, about 5 minutes. Remove from the heat, stir in ½ cup Parmesan, and season with salt and pepper (add extra salt to taste if using water to cook the polenta). Pour into a 9-by-13-inch baking pan, smoothing the top with a rubber spatula, and allow to cool, about 30 minutes. At this point, the polenta can be covered with plastic wrap and refrigerated for up to two days.

2. Bring a large pot of salted water to a boil. Fill a bowl with water and ice. Blanch the broccoli rabe in the boiling water until crisp-tender, about 1 minute. Drain and cool in the ice water. Drain well and chop coarsely.

3. Warm the olive oil in a large pan over medium heat. Add the garlic and cook until fragrant, about 30 seconds. Add the broccoli rabe and red pepper flakes and toss to coat with the oil. Add water and simmer, covered, for 2 minutes. Uncover and continue to simmer if the broccoli rabe is too soupy. Season with salt.

4. Preheat the broiler. Cut the chilled polenta into 6 portions.

5. Lay the polenta on a baking sheet and broil, five inches from the heat source, turning once, until the polenta is golden and slightly crisp on the outside and thoroughly warmed, about 10 minutes.

6. Combine the remaining cup of Parmesan with the mozzarella. Lay the polenta in a large pan and top with the broccoli rabe mixture. Sprinkle the cheese mixture over all and return to the broiler or a covered grill until the cheese is melted and bubbling.

NOTE: You can buy instant polenta in many large supermarkets and gourmet shops. If you can't find it, you can substitute fine yellow cornmeal.

⦿ PEPPERED TUNA WITH RED WINE AND SHALLOTS

Difficulty: Medium-Difficult
Prep Time: 45 minutes
Cook Time: 20 minutes
Servings: 4

Waldy Says: If you are a steak lover, this is the fish dish for you. This sexy steak will be sure to provide you with all of the energy (instead of fat) required for optimum performance. It is essentially steak au poivre, but in this case the steaks are tuna. Like its beef counterpart, the fish is coated in a generous black pepper crust and seared until rare or medium-rare. Then I add a potent, syrupy red wine and port sauce that's chockful of crunchy shallots. It all adds up to an easy, fast-cooking recipe with strong, satisfying flavors. Serve it with traditional steak accompaniments, like watercress salad and potatoes.

4 tuna steaks (1¼-inches thick)
Coarse sea salt or kosher salt to taste
2 teaspoons very coarsely ground black pepper
1 cup dry red wine
½ cup port
3 shallots, diced (about ¾ cup)
1 cup cherry tomatoes, halved
2 teaspoons extra-virgin olive oil
Basil sprigs, for garnish (optional)

1. Season the tuna steaks with salt on both sides, then pat the pepper all over them. Wrap in plastic and refrigerate for 1 hour.

2. In a saucepan over medium heat, combine the wine, port, and shallots and bring to a boil. Simmer until syruplike and reduced, about 20 minutes. Keep warm.

3. Position a well-seasoned or lightly oiled cast-iron skillet six inches from the heat source and pre-heat the broiler for 10 minutes. You can also use an oiled, heavy-duty baking pan. Or, light the grill.

4. In the oven: Carefully lay the tuna steaks in the preheated pan and broil until charred around the edges, about 2 minutes. Turn and cook for 2 minutes more for rare, or until done to taste. On the grill: Lightly oil the grill or a grilling basket. Place the tuna on the grill (or use the basket) and cook for 2 to 3 minutes per side for rare, or until done to taste.

5. In a bowl, toss the cherry tomatoes with the olive oil and season with salt and pepper. Use a slotted spoon to mound the shallots on a platter, top with the tuna, and surround with the tomatoes. Drizzle with the red wine–port syrup and garnish with basil sprigs if desired.

℞ASPBERRY CAKE

Difficulty: Medium
Prep Time: 30 minutes
Cook Time: 30 minutes
Servings: 8

Waldy Says: Fragile and delectable raspberries, with their perfumelike fragrance and delightful flavor, need to be handled with care. Think of this pleasurable antioxidant powerhouse as your prelude to fun. It's a very easy cake that produces dramatic results.

Butter for baking pan
1 cup all-purpose flour, plus more for baking pan
1 teaspoon baking powder
¼ teaspoon salt
2 large eggs, separated
1 cup vegetable shortening

1 cup sugar
⅓ cup milk
1 teaspoon vanilla extract
1 cup raspberries, plus more for serving
Ice cream or whipped cream for serving

1. Preheat the oven to 375°F. Grease and flour a 9-inch-square baking pan. Sift together 1 cup flour, baking powder, and salt.

2. Beat the egg whites with an electric mixer and set them aside. With the same beaters in another bowl, beat the shortening with the sugar; beat in the egg yolks. Alternately add the milk and dry ingredients to the shortening mixture. Fold in the egg whites and vanilla. Add the raspberries and pour the mixture into the pan.

3. Bake for 25 to 30 minutes, until a toothpick inserted in the center comes out dry (except for the raspberry juice!).

4. Put a slice of cake on each plate. Add a scoop of ice cream or a dollop of whipped cream. Sprinkle a few raspberries around the plate.

《MENU TWO   (see page 189)

VENISON CHOPS WITH SPICY CURRANT AND RED WINE SAUCE

Roasted Butternut Squash and Pear Soup
Venison Chops with Spicy Currant
and Red Wine Sauce
Apple Crisps

℞OASTED BUTTERNUT SQUASH AND PEAR SOUP

Difficulty: Medium-Difficult
Prep Time: 1 hour
Cook Time: 45 minutes
Servings: 6

Waldy Says: This succulent spicy soup will inspire all sorts of visions of a chilly evening under covers—the ingredients are formulated to assist you while you are there. Although you might think that the pear, squash, and crystallized ginger would make for a pretty sweet soup, dry white wine and spicy fresh ginger temper this tendency. Instead, the flavors are savory and mellow with a hint of spices, while the garnish of candied ginger adds just the right spark.

1 large butternut squash (about 3 pounds), peeled, seeded, and cut into 1-inch pieces
2 carrots, peeled and cut into 1-inch pieces
1 tablespoon extra-virgin olive oil
Coarse sea salt or kosher salt to taste
Freshly ground black pepper to taste
3 leeks, white and light green parts only, cleaned and sliced
2 Bosc pears, peeled and cut into 1-inch pieces
½ cup white wine
¼ cup brandy
7 cups chicken or vegetable broth (low-sodium if canned), or water
1 large sprig fresh thyme, plus additional leaves for garnish
1-inch piece ginger root, peeled and grated
1 tablespoon chopped crystallized ginger, for garnish

1. Preheat the oven to 450°F. Place the squash and carrots in a roasting pan large enough to hold them in one layer (or use two), and toss with the oil and salt and pepper. Roast for 10 minutes, then add the leeks and pears. Toss to combine and continue to roast for another 30 minutes, until the vegetables are tender and browned.

2. Remove the pan from the oven and immediately add the wine and brandy, using a wooden spoon to scrape the vegetables and their caramelized juices from the sides and bottom of the pan. Transfer the vegetables and liquid to a large soup pot. Pour in the broth or water—adding additional water if necessary—to cover the vegetables by 1 inch. Add the thyme sprig and grated ginger root and bring the liquid to a boil. Reduce the heat and simmer, partially covered, for 1 hour.

3. Remove the thyme sprig and purée the soup either with an immersion blender, or in batches in a blender or food processor. Transfer the soup to a medium-mesh sieve set over another pot. Use a rubber spatula to press the solids through the sieve. If the soup seems too thick, thin it with a little water. Season with salt and pepper.

4. Just before serving, warm the soup over low heat. Serve in warmed bowls and garnish with the crystallized ginger and a sprinkling of fresh thyme leaves.

VENISON CHOPS WITH SPICY CURRANT AND RED WINE SAUCE

Difficulty: Medium-Difficult
Prep Time: 45 minutes
Cook Time: 30 minutes
Servings: 4

Waldy Says: You—the big hunter—serve game that is naturally low in fat and very tasty. I have added circulation-enhancing ingredients. Whether you shoot the deer yourself or know the hunter who did, or if you order it from a fancy catalogue (see note below), you'll want a nice recipe for the chops, since they're the most special part. Venison chops should be cooked like lamb chops, kept rare to medium-rare. Here I coat them in cracked black pepper and add a spicy currant and red wine sauce that's a perfect foil for the pleasantly gamey flavor of venison. Always assume the role of the hunter/provider.

8 venison chops, cut from a rack (about 2 pounds) (see note)

2 tablespoons cracked black peppercorns,
   or to taste
Coarse sea salt or kosher salt to taste
¾ cup dry red wine
2 tablespoons diced shallots
2 cups good quality red or black currant jelly
   or preserves
Watercress sprigs, for garnish

1. Rub the chops on both sides with 1 tablespoon of the peppercorns and salt to taste. Wrap in plastic and let rest at room temperature for 30 minutes or refrigerate for 2 to 4 hours.

2. Light the grill. In a saucepan over medium heat, combine the red wine, shallots, and the remaining tablespoon of peppercorns. Bring to a boil and simmer until syrupy and almost dry, about 12 minutes. Add the currant jelly, reduce the heat to low, and cook until the jelly has melted. Raise the heat and simmer for 3 minutes. Strain the sauce into a serving bowl.

3. Place the chops on the grill and cook for 2 to 3 minutes per side for rare.

4. Serve the venison with the sauce, garnished with watercress sprigs.

NOTE: If you can't find venison chops or a rack near where you live, you can mail order it from D'Artagnan (1-800-327-8246).

½ cup flour
¼ cup cornmeal
2 large apples, peeled and cut into small dice
   (about 1½ cups)
1½ cup white wine
2 tablespoons freshly squeezed lemon juice
2 tablespoons sour cream
Ice cream or whipped cream to serve

1. Preheat oven to 350°F. Combine ¼ cup sugar, butter, flour, and cornmeal in a food processor, pulsing until crumbly. Spread the streusel on a sheet pan and bake at 325°F for 25 minutes or until golden brown. (The mixture will seem to break down and then brown.) Let cool slightly and then crumble into small pieces.

2. Cook the apples, wine, lemon juice, and the remaining ½ cup sugar over medium heat, stirring continuously until the water evaporates and the sugar begins to turn light golden brown. Remove from the heat, let cool 10–15 minutes, add the sour cream, and mix thoroughly.

3. In a 9-inch-square brownie pan, press the streusel into an even layer. Spread the apple mixture over the streusel. Bake for 25–30 minutes. Cut into 4 to 6 squares and serve with ice cream or whipped cream.

APPLE CRISPS

Difficulty:	Easy-Medium
Prep Time:	30 minutes
Cook Time:	30 minutes
Servings:	4

Waldy Says: The original forbidden fruit. Use it to your advantage.

¾ cup sugar
½ cup unsalted butter, diced

WEEK SIX

◖◗MENU ONE   (see page 206)

SWORDFISH STEAKS IN A MUSTARD SEED CRUST

Butter Lettuce Salad with Red Pepper Vinaigrette
Swordfish Steaks in a Mustard Seed Crust
Poached Pears with Apricots and Almonds

BUTTER LETTUCE SALAD WITH RED PEPPER VINAIGRETTE

Difficulty: Easy
Prep Time: 30 minutes
Cook Time: 10 minutes
Servings: 4

Waldy Says: This roasted red pepper vinaigrette is so delicious and intense that you'll want to just dip bread in it and eat it all by itself. Leftovers have a lot of wonderful uses, from topping grilled vegetables or potatoes to marinating chicken or fish, or using as a dip. Here, I pair the vinaigrette with an assortment of light, crunchy vegetables, including tender lettuce, strips of red peppers, and crisp cucumbers. The clean, bright sweetness of this salad really perks up the appetite and libido.

2 red bell peppers
½ cup extra-virgin olive oil, plus additional for brushing the peppers
3 tablespoons sherry or white wine vinegar
1 tablespoon chopped shallot
½ teaspoon coarse sea salt or kosher salt, plus additional to taste
¼ teaspoon freshly ground black pepper, plus additional to taste
1 large head butter lettuce, washed, spun dry, and torn
1 cup flat leaf parsley
1 cucumber, peeled, halved, seeded, and sliced
2 ounces crumbled feta cheese, for garnish (optional)
2 scallions, trimmed and thinly sliced, for garnish (optional)

1. Preheat the broiler.
2. Halve one of the peppers lengthwise and discard the seeds and stem. Lay the pepper skin side up on a baking sheet, brush lightly with olive oil, and place di-rectly under the heat source. Broil until the skin is charred and blistered all over, about 3 minutes.

3. Immediately transfer the pepper to a deep bowl and cover with a plate to trap the steam. Let steam until cool, about 5 minutes, then rub the peel off the pepper using your hands or a metal spoon. Coarsely chop the pepper.

4. In the bowl of a blender or food processor, combine the roasted pepper, vinegar, and shallots. Purée until smooth. With the motor running, slowly drizzle in olive oil. Season with salt and pepper.

5. Seed the remaining pepper and cut it crosswise into very thin strips.

6. Place the lettuce in a salad bowl. Toss with the parsley and cucumber, drizzle with ½ cup vinaigrette, and toss to lightly coat. Garnish the salad with pepper strips, feta, and scallions if desired.

SWORDFISH STEAKS IN A MUSTARD SEED CRUST

Difficulty: Easy
Prep Time: 15 minutes
Cook Time: 15 minutes
Servings: 4

Waldy Says: A powerful dish with flavor to spare. Garnish with some capers for an extra kick. Olive oil, mustard, lemon, and pepper with all the benefits of a great fish should set the stage for a stellar experience.

½ cup Dijon-style mustard
½ cup whole grain mustard
⅛ cup extra-virgin olive oil
3 tablespoons freshly squeezed lemon juice
¼ teaspoon freshly ground black pepper
4 skinless swordfish medallions (1½ to 2 inches thick)
Chopped fresh dill, for garnish (optional)
2 tablespoons capers, for garnish (optional)

1. In a bowl, whisk together the mustards, olive oil, lemon juice, and pepper. Lay the swordfish in a pan in a single layer. Pour some of the mustard mixture over the fish, turning to coat both sides. Cover and refrigerate for at least 20 minutes and up to 2 hours.

2. Preheat the broiler.

3. Lay the fish on a baking sheet about 4 inches from the broiler and cook for 5 minutes. Turn the fish, brush the tops with some of the remaining mustard mixture, and cook for another 10 minutes. Turn once again, brush tops with more mustard mixture, and cook until no longer pink in the middle, about 5 minutes more.

4. Garnish the swordfish with dill and capers if desired.

POACHED PEARS WITH APRICOTS AND ALMONDS

Difficulty: Medium
Prep Time: 30 minutes
Cook Time: 30 minutes
Servings: 4

Waldy Says: The texture and warmth of the poached pears with the flavor of the apricots and almond paste are extremely sensual. Allow the combination to fill your mouth and mind with visions and shapes to lift your libido.

4 large semi-ripe pears, peeled
1 cup Sauternes or other dessert wine
Pulp and pod of 1 vanilla bean
¼ cup freshly squeezed lemon juice
1 cup chopped pitted dried apricots (chopped fine) reconstituted in 1 cup hot water
½ cup almond paste
¼ cup crème fraîche or sour cream
½ cup freshly squeezed orange juice
⅛ teaspoon ground cinnamon

1. Scoop out the core and part of the flesh from the bottom of the pears. Place the pears in a medium-size roasting pan with the Sauternes, vanilla pulp and pod, lemon juice, and enough water to cover the pears. Simmer for 20 minutes or until the tip of a sharp knife inserted into a pear slides out easily. Remove the pears from the liquid and set upright on a towel to cool and drain.

2. Combine ½ cup apricots, almond paste, and crème fraîche and spoon into the cavities of the cooked pears.

3. Combine the remaining ½ cup apricots, orange juice, and cinnamon in a food processor and pulse until smooth. Warm just before serving.

4. Spoon the warm sauce into the center of each plate. Cut each of the pears in half lengthwise and place two halves upright on each plate.

⟲MENU TWO   (see page 206)

CHICKEN BREAST WITH MUSTARD, ALMONDS, AND THYME

Tuna Carpaccio with Basil and Arugula
Chicken Breast with Mustard, Almonds, and Thyme
Blueberry Cobbler

TUNA CARPACCIO WITH BASIL AND ARUGULA

Difficulty: Medium
Prep Time: 30 minutes
Cook Time: 10 minutes
Servings: 4 as a main course

Waldy Says: Carpaccio is a classic Italian appetizer of thinly sliced raw beef, often served with arugula salad and Parmesan cheese. In my version, I substitute sushi-quality tuna for the beef and give the outer edges a slight char on the grill. This lends a rich, smoky flavor to the fish without cooking it through. Bitter arugula and mushrooms round out the flavors, making this dish almost a salad, but substantial enough for a main course.

½ cup packed fresh basil leaves, plus additional sprigs for garnish
7 tablespoons, plus 1 teaspoon extra-virgin olive oil
1 teaspoon coarse sea salt or kosher salt, plus additional to taste
Freshly ground black pepper to taste
10 ounces "grade A" sushi-quality tuna loin
¼ cup dry white wine
2 cups coarsely chopped arugula
4 large white mushroom caps, thinly sliced
1 teaspoon freshly squeezed lemon juice
Shaved Parmesan cheese, for garnish

1. Chop enough of the basil to yield 1 tablespoon. Combine it in a shallow bowl or rimmed plate with 1 teaspoon olive oil and salt and pepper to taste. Add the tuna and turn until well coated. Cover with plastic and refrigerate for 1 hour.

2. Lightly oil the grill basket and light the grill.

3. Meanwhile, in the bowl of a blender or food processor, combine the remaining basil leaves, 4 tablespoons olive oil, white wine, salt, and pepper. Blend basil oil until smooth.

4. Grill tuna for 1 to 2 minutes per side, charring the outside while keeping the center cold and red. Transfer to a board and let cool, then wrap the tuna in plastic and refrigerate for 1 hour or freeze for 20 minutes. This allows the fish to firm up enough to be sliced very thinly. Transfer the tuna to a board and slice as thinly as possible.

5. In a bowl, toss the arugula with 2 tablespoons olive oil. In another bowl, toss the mushrooms with remaining tablespoon of olive oil, the lemon juice, and salt and pepper to taste. Mound some arugula

in the center of each plate and surround it with slices of tuna. Scatter the mushrooms over all, drizzle with some of the basil oil, and garnish with shaved Parmesan and basil sprigs.

CHICKEN BREAST WITH MUSTARD, ALMONDS, AND THYME

Difficulty: Medium
Prep Time: 30 minutes
Cook Time: 30 minutes
Servings: 4

Waldy Says: What may at first seem like an unusual combination of mustard and almonds becomes a crisp, tasty crust that rivals the crunch of fried chicken. The ingredients, almost biblical, conjure up thoughts of vestal virgins and Roman orgies. Using chicken breasts on the bone ensures that the meat will stay moist and flavorful as the skin browns.

¼ cup whole grain mustard
¼ cup Dijon-style mustard
2 tablespoons finely chopped fresh thyme leaves, plus additional sprigs for garnish
¼ teaspoon freshly ground black pepper, plus more to taste
2 tablespoons water
¼ cup extra-virgin olive oil
3 whole chicken breasts, bone-in, skin-on
Coarse sea salt or kosher salt to taste
½ cup sliced natural almonds, toasted (see sidebar), for garnish

1. In a very large bowl, whisk together the mustards, thyme, pepper, and water. Whisk in the olive oil. Place the chicken breasts in the bowl and toss to coat. Cover the bowl and let sit at room temperature for 30 minutes or refrigerate for 2 hours or overnight.

2. Preheat the oven to 500°F. Rinse the chicken

and pat dry with paper towels. Season the chicken with salt and pepper.

3. Lay the chicken breasts skin side down in a roasting pan. Roast for about 25 minutes, turning once and basting with marinade, until the chicken is crisp and cooked through.

4. To serve, halve the chicken breasts, remove and discard the skin, and serve them garnished with the almonds and thyme sprigs and sprinkled with salt.

TOASTING ALMONDS

An easy way to toast almonds is on top of the stove in a skillet. Spread ½ cup almonds in a large skillet and place over high heat. Cook, stirring constantly, until the nuts are fragrant and browned, about 3 minutes. Immediately pour the almonds onto a plate to stop the cooking.

BLUEBERRY COBBLER

Difficulty: Easy
Prep Time: 20 minutes
Cook Time: 35 minutes
Servings: 6

Waldy Says: Blueberries are rich with antioxidants and here is a delicious way to add to your arsenal.

4 to 5 cups blueberries
½ cup, plus 2 tablespoons sugar
1½ tablespoons quick cooking tapioca
9 tablespoons unsalted butter
1 cup all-purpose flour
1½ teaspoons baking powder
¼ teaspoon salt
¼ cup milk
1 large egg, lightly beaten
Vanilla ice cream (optional)

1. Toss together blueberries, ½ cup sugar, tapioca, and 1 tablespoon butter in a medium saucepan and set aside for about 10 minutes to moisten the tapioca. Lightly grease a 1½-quart casserole.

2. Meanwhile, stir together the flour, 2 tablespoons sugar, baking powder, and salt. Cut in the remaining 8 tablespoons butter with a pastry blender or two knives. In a separate bowl, combine the milk and egg. Add all at once to the dry ingredients and stir only until combined. Be careful not to over-mix.

3. Preheat the oven to 400°F. Cook the blueberry mixture over low heat, stirring until it comes to a full boil, about 10 minutes. Pour the blueberry mixture into the casserole and spoon the topping over all. Bake for 20 to 25 minutes, until the cobbler is golden brown. Serve warm with vanilla ice cream, if desired.

THE HARDNESS FACTOR
ULTIMATE PRELUDE DINNER

Waldy Says: Each component of this tasting menu has been carefully selected to evoke romance and sensuality while making sure no ingredients exist to slow your circulation. The eroticism of the flavors does not fully reveal itself until the meal has been experienced in its entirety. The rose champagne, which I recommend enjoying throughout the meal, with its color, effervescence, light acidity, and slightly sweet taste, will accentuate both the bold and subtle flavors of the food.

The meal is designed to emulate the very act of making love. The caviar and oysters provide the culinary foreplay leading to a crescendo of bold flavors in the lamb chop and chutney. The warm chocolate cake and roasted apricots provide a comfort zone of warm afterglow. I recommend taking the cherries and grapes, perhaps with a second bottle of champagne, to a most comfortable location to experience the side effects of this menu.

THE GRAND FEAST

◌◉ *Rose Champagne* ◉◌

Osetra Caviar with Brioche Toast Points,
Crème Fraîche, and Chives

Roasted Oysters with Shallots

Lamb Chops with Mint and Garlic Relish

Roasted Carrots with Honey and Black Pepper

Individual Warm Chocolate Cake with Roasted Apricots, Fresh Cherries, and Seedless Red Grapes

Green Tea with Honey and Lemon

OSETRA CAVIAR WITH BRIOCHE TOAST POINTS, CRÈME FRAÎCHE, AND CHIVES

Caviar is one of the world's most sensuous and romantic foods. Caviar as a prelude to a grand meal sets the tone for the evening. Caviar requires very little additional fuss or preparation. You are limited only by the quality, type, and quantity you purchase. I suggest osetra caviar because it is usually a better value and has great flavor. Always buy caviar fresh and from a reputable source. The caviar should glisten and appear to be individual eggs with absolutely no fish odor. American caviar is available and can be quite good. You should taste it. I recommend at least an ounce per person.

Serve it with toast made from brioche (any good quality bread will do), a dollop of crème fraîche, chopped chives, and a little squeeze of lemon. If you cannot find crème fraîche, sour cream may be substituted. If you like, you can add traditional garnishes of chopped hard cooked eggs and chopped onions. For optimum presentation and appeal, serve the caviar on crushed ice with garnishes surrounding it on individual small plates. The only utensil needed is a caviar spoon or nonreactive tool to spread the caviar on the toast.

In between sips of champagne, savor the caviar as it fills your mouth with the fresh and true flavors of the sea. Take your time. Prepare the toast points and feed each other if you like.

ROASTED OYSTERS WITH SHALLOTS

Difficulty:	Easy
Prep Time:	45 minutes
Cook Time:	15 minutes
Servings:	4

Waldy Says: These oysters are topped with little spoonfuls of a shallot/white wine/butter sauce, which mixes with the oyster juices and reduces in the oven, while the shallots get crisp. Six oysters make an impressive appetizer, or you can pass the oysters still in their baking dish (wear oven mitts) as an hors d'oeuvre. To keep the oysters balanced while they roast, I line the baking dish with a layer of rock salt dotted with peppercorns. The rumors hold true about the benefits of eating oysters—warm ones are just that much more seductive.

3 tablespoons extra-virgin olive oil
1 cup thinly sliced shallots
¼ cup dry white wine or dry vermouth
Coarse sea salt or kosher salt to taste
Freshly ground black pepper to taste
¼ cup chicken stock, vegetable broth, or water
3 tablespoons unsalted butter
1 tablespoon chopped fresh shallots
1 tablespoon chopped fresh parsley
Rock salt to roast the oysters on
3 tablespoons black peppercorns
24 oysters (see sidebar)
Lemon wedges, for serving

1. Preheat the oven to 500°F.

2. In a heavy saucepan over medium heat, heat

the olive oil. Reduce the heat to low and add the shallots and wine or vermouth. Cover and cook until most of the liquid is absorbed, about 4 to 5 minutes. Season with salt and pepper, and add chicken stock and butter. Bring to a simmer, then remove from heat and stir in parsley.

3. Cover with rock salt the bottom of an oven-proof baking dish large enough to hold all the oysters. Sprinkle the peppercorns evenly over the salt. Open the oysters, discarding the top shell. Loosen the oysters from the bottom shell, being careful not to spill their juices, and lay them in the baking dish. Stir the shallot mixture and spoon some over each oyster. Roast until the edges of the oysters just begin to curl, about 5 to 8 minutes. Serve on the baking dish with lemon wedges.

BUYING AND SHUCKING OYSTERS

For this recipe, you need to buy live oysters with unblemished shells. When opened, the meat should be pale (its color will vary, but avoid any that are pink), plump, and glossy, and they should smell like fresh seawater. If they smell "off," discard them.

When you get the oysters home, scrub their shells in cold water with a brush. Store them flat on a baking sheet in the refrigerator, covered with a slightly damp paper towel, and use them within two days.

You can have your fishmonger shuck the oysters for you if you plan to use them immediately; just ask him to reserve their juices so you can bring them home. Before roasting, strain the oyster juice and add a teaspoon of the juice to each oyster.

To shuck live oysters yourself, insert a thin bladed knife (or oyster knife) into the joint, or "foot" of the shell, and twist the blade to loosen the shell. Being careful not to spill the liquid, slide the knife along the top of the shell (not deeply enough to cut the oyster). Discard the upper shell and cut through the muscle holding the oyster to the bottom shell.

LAMB CHOPS WITH MINT AND GARLIC RELISH

Difficulty: Easy
Prep Time: 30 minutes
Cook Time: 30 minutes
Servings: 4 to 6

Waldy Says: I prefer to keep my mint jelly for toast and serve my lamb with a gutsy mix of mint, garlic, and pepper. Vinegar gives this bright, heady relish a slight pungency that accents the flavor of simple lamb chops. The recipe comes together so quickly you could make it after work, but because lamb chops are always special, it's also a great dish for entertaining. The herbs and garlic, and the succulence of the lamb, will have your circulation in overdrive.

1 cup chopped fresh mint
3 tablespoons minced fresh garlic
3 tablespoons extra-virgin olive oil
Freshly ground black pepper to taste
12 lamb chops (1½ inches thick)
Coarse sea salt or kosher salt to taste
⅓ cup dry white wine
¾ cup diced red onion
¾ cup diced tomato
2 teaspoons freshly squeezed lemon juice

1. In a bowl, combine ⅓ cup mint, 1 tablespoon garlic, 2 tablespoons olive oil, and a large pinch of black pepper.

2. Season the chops generously on both sides with salt. Spread the mint-garlic mixture over both sides of the chops and wrap tightly in plastic. Let marinate for 30 minutes at room temperature or refrigerate for at least 4 hours or overnight.

3. Light the grill or preheat the broiler. In a small saucepan over medium heat, combine 2 tablespoons garlic, 1 tablespoon olive oil, and white wine. Bring the mixture to a boil and simmer until almost dry, about 4 minutes. Let cool.

4. In a bowl, combine the cooled garlic mixture with ⅔ cup mint, red onion, tomato, lemon juice, and salt and pepper to taste.

5. On the grill: Lay the chops on the grill and cook, turning once, until it is done to taste, about 3 to 5 minutes per side for medium-rare. In the oven: Lay the chops on a baking pan and place it as close to the heat source as possible. Broil, turning once, until the meat is done to taste, about 3 to 5 minutes per side for medium-rare.

6. Serve the chops immediately with the relish.

ROASTED CARROTS WITH HONEY AND BLACK PEPPER

Difficulty: Easy
Prep Time: 15 minutes
Cook Time: 45 minutes
Servings: 4

Waldy Says: This recipe turns the commonplace, humble carrot into a unique, full-flavored side dish. A generous amount of black pepper gives it spark and vibrancy, while the honey becomes a lacquered glaze that accentuates the sweetness of the carrots. All the ingredients combine into a vitamin for the bloodstream. It is up to you to direct that blood flow to the right place.

    1 large bunch carrots (about 2 pounds), peeled
        and cut diagonally into 1-inch slices
    1 tablespoon unsalted butter, melted
    ¼ teaspoon coarse sea salt or kosher salt, plus
        additional to taste
    ¼ teaspoon fresh, coarsely ground black pepper,
        plus additional to taste
    ½ cup honey
    1 orange, zested and juiced

1. Preheat the oven to 475°F. In a large bowl, toss the carrots with the butter and season with salt and liberal grindings of coarse black pepper. Lay the carrots out in a single layer on rimmed baking sheets and roast until they are browned and almost tender, about 30 minutes.

2. Meanwhile, in a saucepan over medium heat, combine the honey, orange zest and juice, and pepper. Bring to a simmer and cook for 1 minute. Season with salt to taste.

3. Transfer the carrots to a casserole or gratin dish and pour the honey mixture over them. Return the carrots to the oven and roast, uncovered, stirring once, until brown and caramelized, about 8 minutes.

INDIVIDUAL WARM CHOCOLATE CAKES WITH ROASTED APRICOTS, FRESH CHERRIES, AND SEEDLESS RED GRAPES

I am assuming you have tried the Warm Chocolate Cake with Roasted Apricots in Week Three **(page 298)** and the Almond Ricotta Cake with Moscato Roasted Apricots **(page 302)** in Week Four. We are going to combine these two recipes and serve them together with a dollop of whipped cream.

Prepare the apricots ahead of time and keep them warm while you are having dinner. Follow the Warm Chocolate Cake recipe. Place the cakes in the oven 10 minutes before you would like to serve dessert. Prepare the whipped cream in advance and store in the refrigerator. Invert the cakes onto the plates, place two or three apricots beside each, drizzle with apricot syrup, and place a spoonful of whipped cream on top. Serve and enjoy.

I have gotten you this far, and you are on your own from here. Good luck and have fun.

Waldy

THE HARDNESS FACTOR

SIX-WEEK PROGRAM GUIDE>>>>>>>>>>>

Increasing penile hardness is not the only reason why you are going to adhere to the Hardness Factor Six-Week Program. Hardness is just the start; you will also be enhancing your sex life and your relationship with your partner.

In addition, you are going to bolster your health and increase your endurance, strength, flexibility, and vitality. The promise of a harder body and better sex life is certainly worth forty-two days of effort.

After all, hard is good; harder is better.

	WEEK 1	COMPLETED
EXERCISE	Walk 5,000 steps daily Side Lunge Reach (10X each leg) **(see page 88)** Classic Push-Ups (3 sets/3 reps) **(see page 88)** *or* Modified Push-Ups (3 sets/5 reps) **(see page 88)** Plank (30 seconds/3X) **(see page 89)**	
SUPPLEMENT	Pycnogenol (80 mg) + L-arginine (3 g)	
NUTRITION	Reduce portion size by 500 calories/day SPECIAL MEALS Herb-Crusted Salmon **(see page 286)** Sea Scallops **(see page 288)**	
PROJECT	Check the medicine cabinet Doctor visit: physical and blood tests	

	WEEK 2	COMPLETED

EXERCISE	**W**alk 6,000 steps daily
	
	Side Lunge Reach (10X each leg) **(see page 88)**
	Angry Cat Stretch (3X) **(see page 120)**
	Classic Push-Ups (3 sets/5 reps) **(see page 88)**
	   or Modified Push-Ups (3 sets/8 reps)
	   (see page 88)
	Plank (30 seconds/3X) **(see page 89)**
	Cobra (30 seconds/10X) **(see page 120)**	

SUPPLEMENT	**P**ycnogenol (80 mg) + **L**-arginine (3 g); **H**orny Goat Weed (2 500 mg capsules)	
NUTRITION	**D**rink tea **R**educe polyunsaturated fats in diet and replace with monounsaturated fats SPECIAL MEALS **S**ummer Vegetable Risotto **(see page 290)** **C**hili-Rubbed Chicken Fingers **(see page 292)** **R**educe portion size by 500 calories/day	
PROJECT	**R**educe stress in your life; **S**top or reduce smoking	

	WEEK 3	COMPLETED

EXERCISE	**W**alk 7,000 steps daily
	
	Side Lunge Reach (10X each leg) **(see page 88)**
	Angry Cat Stretch (3x) **(see page 120)**
	Woodchopper Exercise (10X) **(see page 146)**
	Classic Push-Ups (3 sets/8 reps) **(see page 88)**
	   or Modified Push-Ups (3 sets/10 reps)
	    (see page 88)
	Plank (45 seconds/3X) **(see page 89)**
	Cobra (10X) **(see page 120)**
	Squat (10X) **(see page 146)**	

SUPPLEMENT	**P**ycnogenol (80 mg) + **L**-arginine (3 g); **H**orny Goat Weed (2 500 mg capsules); **2** Omega-3 fatty acid capsules	
NUTRITION	**A**dd more vegetables to meals **E**at more fruit SPECIAL MEALS **T**urkey Paillards **(see page 294)** **H**alibut with Lemon Confit **(see page 297)** **P**eppered Tuna **(see page 299)**	
PROJECT	**C**ut back on daily alcohol consumption **P**erform a testicle self-exam	

	WEEK 4	COMPLETED

EXERCISE	**W**alk 8,000 steps daily
	
	Side Lunge Reach (15X each leg) **(see page 88)**
	Angry Cat Stretch (3X) **(see page 120)**
	Woodchopper Exercise (15X) **(see page 146)**
	Bridge (10X) **(see page 168)**
	Classic Push-Ups (3 sets/8 reps) **(see page 88)**
	   or Modified Push-Ups (3 sets/10 reps)
	   (see page 88)
	Plank (45 seconds/4X) **(see page 89)**
	Cobra (10X) **(see page 120)**
	Squat (15X) **(see page 146)**
	Squat Thrust (3X) **(see page 168)**	

SUPPLEMENT	**P**ycnogenol (80 mg) + **L**-arginine (3 g); **H**orny Goat Weed (2 500 mg capsules); **2** Omega-3 fatty acid capsules; **1** 200 mg red wine extract; **1** 100 mg grape seed extract	
NUTRITION	**A**dd fish to the weekly menu **SPECIAL MEALS** **R**oasted Shellfish Stew **(see page 301)** **C**risp Penne **(see page 303)**	
PROJECT	**P**ull the plug on your TV **I**ncrease the amount of sleep time	

	WEEK 5	COMPLETED
EXERCISE	Walk 9,000 steps daily Side Lunge Reach (15X each leg) **(see page 88)** Angry Cat Stretch (3X) **(see page 120)** Woodchopper Exercise (20X) **(see page 146)** Bridge (15X) **(see page 168)** Hip-Flexor Stretch (Hold 15 seconds each leg) **(see page 194)** Classic Push-Ups (3 sets/10 reps) **(see page 88)** Plank (60 seconds/4X) **(see page 89)** Cobra (10X) **(see page 120)** Squat (20X) **(see page 146)** Squat Thrust (5X) **(see page 168)** Single-Leg Squat (5X each leg) **(see page 194)**	
SUPPLEMENT	Pycnogenol (80 mg) + L-arginine (3 g); Horny Goat Weed (2 500 mg capsules); 2 Omega-3 fatty acid capsules; 1 200 mg red wine extract; 1 100 mg grape seed extract; 2 400 mg niacin capsules	
NUTRITION	Make a commitment to eat breakfast daily Add soy protein to the diet Cut back on meat **SPECIAL MEALS** Peppered Tuna **(see page 305)** Venison Chops **(see page 307)**	
PROJECT	Reduce stress in your life Stop smoking Don't weigh yourself daily Determine your BMR Learn how to maximize sperm production	

	WEEK 6	COMPLETED

EXERCISE	**W**alk 10,000 steps daily
	
	Side Lunge Reach (15X each leg) **(see page 88)**
	Angry Cat Stretch (4X) **(see page 120)**
	Woodchopper Exercise (20X) **(see page 146)**
	Single Leg Bridge (5X each leg) **(see page 216)**
	Hip-Flexor Stretch (15 seconds/each leg)
	   (see page 194)
	Neck Stretch (4X) **(see page 216)**
	Classic Push-Ups (3 sets/10 reps) **(see page 88)**
	Plank (60 seconds/5X) **(see page 89)**
	Cobra (10X) **(see page 120)**
	Squat (20X) **(see page 194)**
	Squat Thrust with Push-Ups (5X) **(see page 168)**
	Single-Leg Squat (5X each leg/no chair)
	   (see page 194)
	Back Extension (5X) **(see page 216)**
	Child's Pose (60 seconds) **(see page 217)**	

SUPPLEMENT	**P**ycnogenol (80 mg) + **L**-arginine (3 g); **H**orny Goat Weed (2 500 mg capsules); **2** Omega-3 fatty acid capsules; **1** 200 mg red wine extract; **1** 100 mg grape seed extract; **2** 400 mg niacin capsules; **1** 500 mg vitamin C; **1** 400 IU vitamin E	
NUTRITION	**E**at smaller lunches and dinners **E**at blueberries SPECIAL MEALS **S**wordfish Steaks **(see page 309)** **C**hicken Breast **(see page 311)** **U**ltimate Prelude Dinner **(see page 313)**	
PROJECT	**S**et aside time for daily contemplation	

EQUIPMENT

OUR SHOPPING LIST

Over the past few years, I have noted a mushrooming of enthusiasm among my patients for dietary supplements. With few peer-reviewed clinical studies to back up claims of efficacy, many now take potions, mixtures, and extracts on their own to self-treat or prevent everything from lagging libido, the common cold, headaches, arthritis, and anxiety to high cholesterol and prostate distress. Some of these supplements can affect the body in ways similar to prescription medications.

Before continuing, let's first deal with nomenclature. Since so many terms are bandied about nowadays and often used interchangeably, from herbal supplement to vitamin and mineral supplement, let's clear the air about what exactly constitutes a dietary supplement. For my way of thinking, a dietary supplement is any product that supplements the diet and contains one or more of the following ingredients: a mineral, vitamin, amino acid, or an herb or other botanical, which can be a plant or plant part valued for its medicinal qualities.

Dietary supplements are valued the world over and play a significant role in primary healthcare in many countries. Billions of dollars are spent annually in the United States for these supplements, but since they are not considered drugs as a result of the Dietary Supplement Health and Education Act of 1994, they are not regulated by the FDA. However, the establishment of the National Center for Complementary and Alternative Medicine, in response to the public demand for information, currently functions as a source for information.

With no laboratory testing of dietary supplements required, we don't really know if a particular supplement has any health benefit, nor do we have any guarantee of potency, purity, or safety. Instead, we put our trust in the dietary supplement industry and assume that the supplements listed on the label are actually in the containers.

Caveat Emptor

It's important that people understand that many dietary supplements, while they are dilute drugs, are still drugs containing active compounds with the possibility of interacting, sometimes antagonistically, within your body.

Be smart and safe. Alert your doctor to what you're taking and how much and how often. Ask if you can take the supplement with other medicines and be sure to find out if you need to avoid certain foods, beverages, or other products when taking a supplement. Failure to ask may result in unwanted side effects that easily could have been avoided.

Walk into any pharmacy or health food store and you are immediately confronted with aisle after aisle of supplements. Many times there are multiple rows containing competing brands of the same vitamin or mineral. To make things easier for you, I have compiled a list of products and created a Hardness Factor Shopping List. These are products that I am familiar with and are made by companies that I know meet the highest industry standards for purity. In addition to the supplements are manufacturers of step counters and home model body fat scales.

Some of the products are found in your drug store or health food store; others are available through mail order. I have provided addresses, both street and email, so you can contact them for product information or to place an order.

HORNY GOAT WEED
Exotica

Pinnacle
175 Lauman Lane
Hicksville, NY 11801
1-800-899-2749
www.pinnaclebody.com

NIACIN
Res-Q HDL +

N3 Oceanic, Inc.
Palm Industrial Center
1862 A Tollgate Rd.
Palm, PA 18070
1-800-262-5483
www.n3inc.com

OMEGA-3 MARINE OILS
Res-Q 1250

N3 Oceanic, Inc.
Palm Industrial Center
1862 A Tollgate Rd.
Palm, PA 18070
1-800-262-5483
www.n3inc.com

HEART HEALTH SYSTEM

Market America, Inc.
1302 Pleasant Ridge Rd.
Greensboro, NC 27409
1-336-605-0040
www.marketamerica.com

OPC
Isotonix OPC-3
   (red wine extract and grape
   seed extract)

Market America, Inc.
1302 Pleasant Ridge Rd.
Greensboro, NC 27409
1-336-605-0040
www.marketamerica.com

PYCNOGENOL/L-ARGININE
Pycnogenol and L-arginine are
   available at any GNC,
   pharmacy, or health food
   store nationwide.

GNC
300 Sixth Avenue
Pittsburgh, PA 15222
1-800-766-7099
www.gnc.com

Pycnogenol Plus
   (mixture of Pycnogenol and
   L-arginine)

The Vitamin Factory
P.O. Box 278
Hillside, NJ 07205-0278
1-800-619-1199
www.vitafac.com/store/home.asp

Prelox Blue
(mixture of Pycnogenol and
L-arginine)

**Herbalife International of
America, Inc.**
P.O. Box 80210
Los Angeles, CA 90080-0210
1-866-866-4744
www.herbalife.com

and

GNC
300 Sixth Avenue
Pittsburgh, PA 15222
1-800-766-7099
www.gnc.com

BODY FAT SCALES
Tanita BF 593 Family Model

**Tanita Corporation of America,
Inc.**
2625 South Clearbrook Drive
Arlington Heights, IL 60005

1-800-TANITA-8
www.tanita.com

STEP COUNTERS
Accusplit Eagle 120 XL

Accusplit
2290A Ringwood Ave.
San Jose, CA 95131
1-800-935-1996
www.accusplit.com

Yamax Digiwalker SW-200
1-888-748-5377
www.store.yahoo.com/
n-e-wlifestyles/digstepcoun.html

Additional information
about the Hardness Factor
Program, including tips,
exercises, and an assortment
of products can be found at
www.thehardnessfactor.com.

VISUAL AID

HEALTH CLASS REDUX

It's like all relationships: We have a comfortable sense of our penis as a friend but we don't usually want to know how all of it works—it's just male magic. But part of our evolution as men is dealing with what makes it all work. So, here for you is a road map of your friend, the penis.

ATLAS OF THE PENIS

PROSTATE GLAND

URINARY BLADDER

CORPORA CAVERNOSA

PROSTATE URETHRA

BULBOURETHRAL GLAND

CORPUS SPONGIOSUM

SPONGY URETHRA

MEMBRANOUS URETHRA

GLANS PENIS

SCROTUM

EXTERNAL URETHRAL ORIFICE

JONNY COHEN

(NOT ACTUAL SIZE)

BIOGRAPHIES

STEVEN LAMM, M.D.

Dr. Lamm, a graduate of Columbia University and New York University School of Medicine, is an internist with a private medical practice in New York City. For the past ten years, Dr. Lamm has regularly reported on a variety of medical issues on local and national television and radio, offering his analysis and help on medical topics. He has been the long-time medical correspondent for *The View* (ABC-TV) because of his ability to talk to women about their important health issues, and the health issues of the men they love.

Dr. Lamm is active in clinical research and has served as an investigator for several sexual medicine studies. He is also a popular lecturer, an educator of doctors, and a visiting professor for numerous pharmaceutical companies. He lives in New York City with his wife and five children. This is Dr. Lamm's fourth book.

Financial Disclosure: Dr. Lamm has received research grants, served as a visiting professor or advisor for, or has received travel expenses from Pfizer, Lilly-ICOS, Solvay, Bayer, Sanofi-Aventis, Horphag, Pinnacle, and N3 Oceanic.

GERALD SECOR COUZENS

A noted contributor to several medical newsletters, he has coauthored more than twenty-four health and medical books. He lives in New York City with his wife and four children.

WALDY MALOUF

The chef and co-owner of the Beacon Restaurant & Bar in New York City, he is also the author of two cookbooks, *High Heat* and *The Hudson Valley Cookbook.*

JANA ANGELAKIS

A certified personal trainer, she is the owner of PEx Personalized Exercise, Inc., located in New York City (www.pexinc.com). Since 1989, Jana, a two-time U.S. Olympian and Fencing Hall of Fame Inductee, has provided, along with her team of professionals, personal training services to discerning New Yorkers.

JONNY COHEN

A cartoonist and illustrator whose drawings appear in *The New Yorker, Reader's Digest UK,* several Barnes and Noble cartoon calendars and diaries, and a greeting card line. He lives with his wife on the small coastal island of Manhattan. He pours the undisputed best martini in New York.

SPECIAL NOTE:
Additional information about the Hardness Factor Program, including tips, exercises, and an assortment of products can be found at www.thehardnessfactor.com

Index

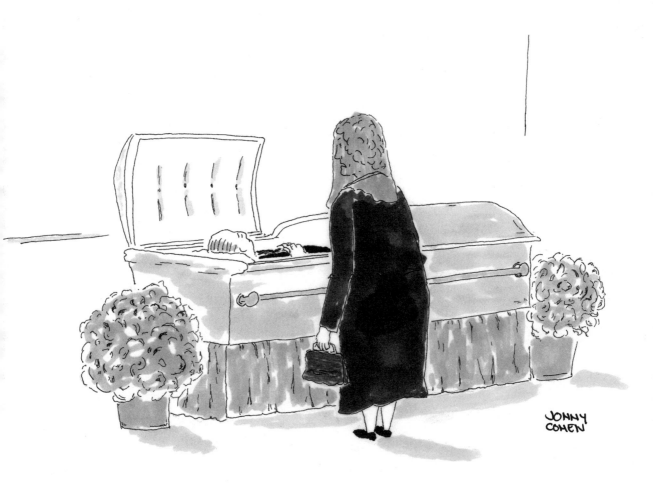

"SO NOW YOU'RE STIFF?"